Copyright 2019

Printed by Kindle Direct Publishing

The views expressed in this work are solely those of the author and do not reflect the views of the publisher.

To obtain copies you may purchase them at Amazon.com

Printed in the United States of America

ISBN: 9781797490625

# DIGNITY

in Living

and

in Dying

## At the Crossing

Love only seems to stop breathing
In that nanosecond
Where time and timeless splash
Into the Everflowing Stream.
We all are caught, gasp -
Pulled along
By love remembered
Newly awakened
Unencumbered.
Free!

Martha Bartholomew

# Dedication

This writing is dedicated to those who have chosen to live life with dignity and wish to consider the possibilities and options for ending their life with dignity.

"If the push towards life sustaining technology were balanced with options for comfort care in both medical school training and the healthcare culture, more people would have the chance to transition to death with dignity and grace."

— Lisa J. Shultz, A Chance to Say Goodbye: Reflections on Losing a Parent

"I lived my whole life following others' wishes. Let me follow my own wish in my death."

— Shon Mehta, The Timingila

# Content

**Dedication**      5

**Acknowledgements**      10

**Preamble "Mt. Evans at Timberline"** 11

**Introduction**      15

**Finish Strong, My Preferences**      17
    -Ralph McFadden

**Part I**

    **What is Dignity?**      19
        A note from Wilbur McFadden

    **Life with Dignity - Being Gay**      21

    **An Excellent Thought on Dignity**      27
        Carol Wise

    **A Contribution – Martha Bartholomew**

Part II

# Entering the Dialogue

A Short Story  -  Ralph McFadden  30
   I Think I May Leave the Party Early

Moses Mason                          39

John Katonah                         46

Richard Baer – a new thought         49
   "Patient Refusal of
      Nutrition and Hydration"

Article by Ira R. Byock              50
   "Patient Refusal of
      Nutrition and Hydration"

Katy Butler - "The Art of Dying Well: A
   Practical Guide to a Good End of
   Life"                             53

Anton van Niekerk,                   60
Anton van Niekerk: Distinguished
Professor of Philosophy and Director: Centre
for Applied Ethics, Stellenbosch University.

NHPCO                                67
   National Hospice and Palliative Care
      Organization
   Statement on Legally Accelerated Death

**Part III**

**The Right to Die – a personal view**  70
**The Chambered Nautilus**  75
**Religion and Spirituality**  78


**Part IV**

**Conclusions**

    **Wherever You Go**  100
    **Richard Baer**  102
    **I'll Be on My Way**  105
    **Crossroads and Choices**  108

**Part V**

**Appendix: Resources** 121

**Legal Aspects**

    **American Public and State Stats** 130

    **Power of Attorney for Health Care** 131

    **Illinois End of Life Options Coalition** 132

    **Final Illinois Options** 133

    **Compassion and Choices** 134

    **Death with Dignity National Center** 139

# Acknowledgements

A very thoughtful and heart-felt thank you to my children for their gracious and loving support: Joel and Laura, and Jill and Anne. My partner, Keo, has been supportive and understanding.

Thank you to the many friends and family who read, considered, and/or contributed to "Dignity": Richard Baer, Martha Bartholomew, Ben Brobst-Renaud, Scott Douglas, Jackie Hartley, Danielle Henson, John Katonah, Cassidy McFadden, Jill McFadden, Anne Tapp, Joel McFadden, Laura McFadden, Rosanna McFadden, Tim McFadden, Wilbur McFadden, Tren Meyers, Michael Novelli, Beat Sauter, Curt Slaybaugh, Katie Shaw-Thompson, Maurice Shenk, Jonathan Shively, and Carol Wise.

And a very grateful thank you to the specific contributors: Richard Baer, Martha Bartholomew, Katy Butler, John Katonah, Shawn Kirchner, Moses Mason, Wilbur McFadden, Michael Novelli, and Anton van Niekerk.

I am thankful, also, to the End of Life Options Coalition, Final Illinois Options, Compassion and Choices, and Death with Dignity National Center for their on-going support for death with dignity advocacy and programs.

# Preamble

## Mt. Evans at Timberline

Mt. Evans at timberline with the grand old
crones and sages—
    survivors, gnarled, fire-scarred, bent
      with the shape
    of the centuries of age and wind,
      among boulders
    coated with gray and green lichen,
    and the tundra, quilted with golden,
      yellow, sky- blue, white, bronze, red,
        and violet—summer
    conquerors of a deadly winter,
    each one amazed at its own returning
      to the land of the living.

All— trees, stones, flowers, grasses—
    perched here within the endless ranges
      of towering
    might and majesty— and with some of
      the granite giants still harboring
    inlets of August snow from last
      spring's heavy pack.
    A mystical place!

I've been here before. Often.
    To sit on grass or needles or rock.
    To know that here on these quiet
        secluded slopes lay the
           ashes of two men—one in his fifties
              and the other in his seventies.

Larry died early—and his family scattered
    his ashes while the bagpipes—
        two hundred yards away, dirging an
           ancient, plaintive mountain melody
           called us to consider our mortality.

And Harold—whose family lived in West
   Virginia—only asked that his wishes for
      his ashes to be scattered
      in the mountains - be carried out
      —and I chose this sacred ground
        because I knew it.

The ground has received the ashes—and two
   winters have sucked them into the arid
      and shallow topsoil.

Two men who lived with family and friends,
   who fashioned their lives around jobs,
   sex, and wonderment about living.

Here I now sit on a hard, unyielding
    boulder, its
        roughness imprinting on my aging
        buttocks—aware—
    but not able to comprehend my own
        finitude,
    my miniscule being in a timeless infinite
        universe.

One day my ashes will join those scattered
    here on this
        ancient peninsula with weathered and
        whitened stones and pines.

One day—how soon? Will my death be
    simply another death and one day—
    there being an energy of Soul
        —will my Light also be free of body -
    and, hopefully, free of this torment of
        uncertain being?

I can't comprehend it—soul without body—
    and what of mind, thinking, feeling?

I retreat to this haven—this place of the
    boundary of tree life at its last—

I retreat—knowing that I am only a few
   seconds away from a road
      battered with tires and tourists and
         noises and yet—
      in the midst of this place—
         the only eternity I presently know.

   Ralph McFadden—1995


The front cover photo is by Ralph McFadden
-   An ancient survivor at 11,000 feet on Mt Evans

# Introduction

In 1991, facing and navigating a midlife career change, I applied for and was accepted into the one-year chaplain residency training program at Rush-St. Luke's Presbyterian Hospital in Chicago. My primary focus for the year was to work with those infected by HIV/AIDS.

After I received my advanced standing as a chaplain, I applied for and was accepted into a full-time chaplain position with Hospice of Metro Denver Hospice, now The Denver Hospice. Ten years later I worked, again as a chaplain, with Journey Care, the not-for-profit hospice and Palliative Care in Northeast Illinois.

My primary responsibility with the hospice program for the first four or five years in Denver was to be a chaplain for many young, gay men dying with AIDS. In that ministry I also worked with patients, partners and families planning for and carrying out memorial services.

It was during the chaplaincy in Metro Denver and Journey Care in Illinois, that I confronted the reality that there were choices when death was close. I learned that very often the patient, the family, and the friends did not understand that there could be options.

In the past few years I have discovered through my reading, journaling, and the death and illnesses of family and friends that there are options that I wish to seriously consider for myself in my final days.

I remember and reflect on the death of Ko, the brother of my partner Keo, and his decisions. Ko and his wife chose to 'fight' even though, with pancreatic cancer, his death was, according to statistics, inevitable. After the diagnosis he lived for 12 months, much of it in pain. He could have chosen to live for 6 months, get comfort care, and could have taken the time to share his love and his gratitude for their support and love. He died in misery with all of the tubes, unable, in the final hours, to communicate or identify his love for his family. Yet, it was his choice and the choice of his family.

I also reflect on my ITP - Immune thrombocytopenia – 18 years now - and then the very recent diagnosis of multiple myeloma. My dad died of multiple myeloma in 1965. He was 59. Medicine for myeloma was in its infancy at that time.

Now meds for myeloma are more advanced. I could still end up with stage four and a lot of pain with this bone cancer. Or I could live another 5 to 8 years with the myeloma in remission.

# Finish Strong – My Preferences
## Ralph McFadden

I am, as I write, keeping in mind the possible choices that I have. I certainly do have preferences.

I will make it clear to Keo, my partner, what those preferences are. I also I want my children - Joel and Jill, to be very clear about my choices in the event of terminal illness. I will share these notes with my primary care physician, my oncologist, my attorney, and the three persons I have identified in "My Power of Attorney for Health Care" as Successor Health Care Agents.

"Finish Strong: Putting Your Priorities First at Life's End" is the title of a book by Barbara Coombs Lee. I will mention more about it in the Appendix section of this book.

Barbara Coombes Lee is the president of Compassion & Choices, a national agency that "improves care, expands options and empowers everyone to chart their end-of-life journey. We envision a society that affirms life and accepts the inevitability of death, embraces expanded options for compassionate dying, and empowers everyone to choose end-of-life care that reflects their values, priorities, and beliefs."

Coombs notes "It's hard to talk about death in America. But even though the topic has been taboo, life's end is an eventual reality."

Coombs makes it clear that we should develop with our loved ones 'advance directives' that specify details about what we want and do not want in the event of terminal illness.

Compassion and Choices offers a booklet entitled *"My End-of-Life Decisions – an Advance Planning Guide and Toolkit"*.

I have read and filled in some of the thirty pages of the Toolkit. I have made copies, shared them with my immediate family and my primary care doctor and oncologist. I have also asked my immediate family if they have questions and to agree that they will support me in my preferences.

From my vantage point, it has been a very helpful process. For further clarification, please check on the internet *"My End-of-Life Decisions: An Advance Planning Guide and Toolkit."* The Toolkit can also be found on the Compassion and Choices website: www.compassion&choices.org.

# Part I

## What is Dignity?

The focus for this writing is "Dignity in Living and Dignity in Dying." For me, dignity is a matter of self-esteem, self-worth, and self-respect. Dignity is self- acceptance and self-actualization.

> "Knowing yourself is the beginning of all wisdom."
> — Aristotle
>
> "The unexamined life is not worth living."
> — Socrates

My friend, Martha Bartholomew shared: "Dignity is that which both *is* and *offers* hospitality to the reality of the moment."

When person **A** treats person **B** with dignity, it means person **A**
acknowledges person **B**'s dignity (worth or value).

## Contributed by Dr. Wilbur McFadden

"Dignity is the right to be treated with respect and to be treated ethically. I don't know how much reflection, as we know it, goes on in the minds of those with Down's Syndrome. But genetically, most have a happy disposition. When I was in practice, I would go to a CME program at Mayo Clinic yearly. One of the lectures one year was by a pediatrician who showed slides of his patients with Downs, and gave them his voice-over, speaking for them. At the end of his lecture, he received a standing ovation from the 300+ physicians---the only such demonstration I could remember out of 400+ lectures. Their dignity, and ALL those with Downs was affirmed!!

So, a definition of dignity should include the many aspects---those we hope for, those we claim for ourselves, and those we bestow on others, whether ethically, morally, legally or politically."

**Dalai Lama wrote:**

"Whether you believe in God or not does not matter so much, whether you believe in Buddha or not does not matter so much, as a Buddhist, whether you believe in reincarnation or not does not matter so much. You must lead a good life. And a good life does not mean good food, good clothes, good shelter. These are not sufficient.

A good motivation is what is needed: compassion without dogmatism, without complicated philosophy; just understanding that others are brothers and sisters and respecting their rights and human dignity."

# Life with Dignity - Being Gay

Author: Ralph McFadden

*Excerpts from the book "For Life is a Journey"*

## I. The Journey

In a book "How, Then, Shall We Live?" by Wayne Muller, he quotes a woman who was taught by her family that she ought to be ashamed because she was not white.

She said, "If we feel ashamed of who we are, we will pretend to be someone else. In the process of trying to satisfy these demands, to be someone else, we do great harm to our natural sense of self. When we struggle to create a new persona that is less offensive and more pleasing, acting the way they want us to be, just to feel safe, acting this way over and over and over, each day, year after year - in time we begin to forget who we are."

In 1969 I "came out" as a gay man to Barbara, my wife. I do not think that I had expected, as I ventured into this new area of my life, "coming out," that I would experience grief and loss. Perhaps I thought that it would change my life. But what was unexpected was how much it would change my very being.

Barbara and I, one Christmas vacation in the late 70's when son Joel was in graduate school and daughter Jill was at a university, told them that I was bisexual or gay. We were still married, and we stayed together until the mid-90's. And even though I was aware of my sexual desires, I did not act on them, only spoke of them. During the years of the 70's and 80's I told a few friends, then, one Thanksgiving, 1989, I told my extended family.

The primary and most intense focus of 'coming out' to myself and to others was when I was in CPE - a year-long chaplain training residency program in at Rush-Presbyterian-St. Luke's Medical Center in Chicago. That was in 1988-89.

It was then that I began to realize that coming to terms with myself would mean tremendous loss. I said, midway into that year, that I would no longer take a job in which I could not be open if I wished.

I think that I also knew, though it was not spoken, that there was an inevitability about this coming out -- that it would mean something life changing for work, for my marriage and for my family. And that was so.

Although the coming out was a matter of integrity, freedom, and a new and adventuresome path, it was also a matter, over months and years, of loss – of friends, of job possibilities, and even the respect and caring of others.

Following my chaplaincy residency, I was hired as a chaplain with Hospice of Metro Denver. There I began to learn about the nature of grief, its impact, the journey through grief, and the rediscovery of new life. Grief was, for me, intimately related to my own journey.

I also began to learn, working with men, women and children with AIDS -- and with partners, and families, and friends -- of the fear, dread, hostility, and rejection around AIDS and of those who were gay.

I experienced much of that negative response about gays and AIDS from Christians. When that undesirable awareness started, I cannot say precisely, but I began to experience a growing mistrust of and anger with the church.

A part of this anger and grief was the awareness that the church was not behaving like I had expected it to behave. I had been tremendously naive. I am a born and bred Brethren. I had a history with the church believing that it was deeply immersed in justice, reconciliation and peace.

My father and mother taught me about compassion, peace, reconciliation and justice. We had Japanese Americans in our home in the early 40's when it was very unpopular. The church in Troy, Ohio where Dad was pastor was one of the first in the Church of the Brethren to have a "Negro" family as members. My father was on the cutting edge of Open Housing in

Elgin, Illinois in the early 50's when he was pastor there.

I especially learned something about dignity, integrity, openness, compassion, reconciliation and justice when I decided to come out as a gay man to my family, friends, and to the church.

The good thing for me about coming out and being gay was the sad, depressing, dreadful and sometimes overwhelming struggle I have had to go through to become this unique person that I am.

*To be challenged, to come out to oneself, and to come out to others has taken courage, heart, and energy, and has ultimately resulted, for me, in a very high degree of integrity. I have had to learn what it is to be authentic and genuine. I experienced dignity.*

In Muller's book, he writes: "Within the sorrow, there is grace. When we come close to those things which break us down, we touch those things that also break us open."

In coming out, after the first awareness of grief and loss, there has been a middle time in this journey, a time of valuing, of remembering, of bargaining, of ruminating, of cursing, of being stunned, disbelieving, of being incredulous. It can be, and was for me, not only a time of intense feelings of disbelief, agony and pain, but also a time of discovery -- a rethinking about life. Again, experiencing dignity.

In this middle time of reevaluating, and feeling anger, and mistrust, and uncertainty, I was aware of something else Muller said: "How many of us are secretly waiting for some magical permission - like a diagnosis of terminal illness - before we truly begin to listen to the quiet dreams, the desires of the heart?"

In the struggling, the discovering, and the exploring came rebirth, reinvention, reorganizing, and dignity.

To be out is to be strong and to be identified with integrity. Certainly, there is still hurt, loss, and struggle. Yet there is also strength, insight, and affirmation of Self; recognition of Dignity. It is an embracing of my own dignity.

This journey has been, for me, at times, a struggle,
    unreal, unbelievable,
        inconceivable, incredible, incredulous,
       dismaying, shocking, frustrating,
     challenging, powerless and powerful,
    hopeless and hopeful, enslaving, and freeing.

Do you recall the poignant scene in "Philadelphia?" Andy, played by Tom Hanks, dying with AIDS, talking late at night with his attorney, Denzel Washington, holding on to his IV pole, listening to Maria Callas singing about tragedy. Andy is caught in a trance of the soaring music, tears streaming down his face, interpreting the words from the Italian... "For out of sorrow comes love."

*And out of sorrow comes strength, Self, a deepening of spirit and compassion; dignity.*

I am sure that I have not learned enough from the sorrow. I realize that sometimes I have not learned love, or compassion, or deepening of the spirit. I am still on that journey, and it is and will be an endless journey. Yet, for me, it is better to be on the journey than to be sitting permanently in some highway rest area.

Once again, Wayne Muller: "The heart of most spiritual practice is simply this: Remember. Remember who you are. Remember what you love. Remember what is sacred. Remember what is true. Remember that you will die, and that this day is a gift. Remember how you wish to live."

## Another excellent thought on Dignity
### Carol Wise

I like the opening focus upon dignity, and I think I know how you are using that concept. However, I thought one aspect that was lacking was an articulation of a more transcendent understanding of dignity. One thing that many marginalized people have had stripped from them is their inherent dignity as a person of worth. What you describe in your coming out, seems to me to in part be a process of claiming your own dignity, your pride and self-respect as a gay man. As you make clear, that was not an easy journey. It was filled with grief and losses. Yet it also helped to make you a more whole, insightful and authentic person. I do think that working to claim our God-given/inherent/human dignity is a particular and very challenging task that marginalized people have to work at because we have internalized so many social messages that question our inherent worth as a person.


## A Story of Dignity
### Contributed by Ralph McFadden
### Attributed to Martha Bartholomew

My friend, Martha, discovers the heart of dignity in nature, relationships, and circumstance.

Martha and David lived for 38 years in a wooded place, a small arboretum established in the forties by an immigrant Swedish botanist, Torkel Korling, north of an area that was to become a shopping mall in the nineties – Springhill at Dundee, IL.

They both tended the wooded area into a retreat center. One building was a Hermitage. Many came there for silent meditation. Often, they would spend time in conversation with Martha.

Martha and David grew older, of course. Age and illness eventually led the two of them to move into a retirement community that offered independence and as needed health care accessible near-by. A community of dignity.

David, in good company, concluded his earthly journey a little over a year ago.

Over many years, Martha and I have developed our friendship into a remarkable sharing of our life's journey.

Today, before I went to Martha's condo in the retirement home, I noted the visitor signing in before me (we are all asked to do that when we come to see someone), was from JourneyCare, the not-for-profit hospice in our area. The visit was to another resident.

As we visited today, I shared my observation with Martha, she stated the obvious, but not often spoken;

"We are a community of persons on the last part of our journey."

And then she told me something she observes as she participates in the writer's group where she lives. There, among residents, members are encouraged to relive their stories, reflect, sometimes laugh on their way toward integrating life with perhaps new insight. It is a place to pause, listen, a place of dignity, listeners having fun among travelers/writers.

"The writing, from my perspective, is giving dignity not only for living, but also for dying."

Martha's openness is an invitation into a creative awareness of the importance of life before, now and yet to be. Her respect is an act of dignity.

# Part II
## Entering the Dialogue

**A Short Story** by Ralph McFadden

### I Think I May Leave the Party Early

Even before attending the Saturday memorial gathering for my sister-in-law, Joyce, I was tilting toward wondering if nonexistence or oblivion might be a good choice. I was having these recurring daymares — nightmares that kept creeping into my daytime consciousness.

My past career was not helpful. I had been, as a hospice chaplain, assigned to nursing homes where all too often I had observed older men in the hallways, who were frequently hardly living as they moved ever so slowly toward dying. Hospice had made life as pleasant as possible for those who were—as the nurses said — "leaving the pier for the last time."

But it wasn't the dying that bothered me. It was the non-hospice pathetic and aging men who were living and not dying — for instance, Edgar, on hallway four in the Good Samaritan of Life Nursing Home. (Not the actual name.)

When I went to see a patient with hospice, Edgar, a resident, was always there ... in his wheelchair ... just sitting ... bent over, restrained (not tightly) with a belt to keep him from falling out of the chair, a bib on his chest usually stained with the droppings of the last breakfast. He had been fed by a very busy aid who was overwhelmed with too many other "Edgars" to feed. And his diaper hadn't been changed.

But the dirty bib and smelly diaper were not the issue: it was the vivid, crystal clear, and somber reality of an old man who had stroked and was now unable to care for himself, wipe his own ass, feed himself, and who could speak only in a garble. And he was living—if that's what you want to call it—with the possible expectation of being in this condition for years. My nightmare/daymare was that I saw my myself there. It was this vivid daymare that harassed me.

And now—at my sister-in-law's memorial service—I was surrounded by men and women, many my own age, who were attending the memorial service; some a little younger, some a little older, some in decent health, but many in deteriorating mental, spiritual, and physical conditions. I, nearly 80 years old, found myself struggling with the frightening image of myself in a similar condition in another year, or even another month.

Annie, bent almost double with osteoporosis, holding onto her walker, peering up at me through her thick glasses, saying something that when I leaned over to hear but I couldn't make out.

Wayne, still upright, with a grin on his face, calling me by another name because he had me confused with his brother ... a brother who had died two years ago.

Wilma, not bad physical condition, saying hello—and then one minute later, saying hello—and I, knowing that she was in an early stage of Alzheimer's, not comforted by the possibility of such a future.

Zane, still intelligent and yet slightly bent, shuffling with his walker, ever so slowly, to get anywhere.

And there were the ones who could not make it to the service—but I clearly remembered them.

Gene, a friend of past years, who was not here for the service, because he was in a nursing home health care with end-stage lung cancer.

Gerry, confined to her room in the health care center with a feeding tube leading into her abdomen, keeping her just barely alive, but neither Gerry nor her family wanted to give up. And toting an ostomy bag on her side because her intestine was no longer functioning. I knew the experience from past surgeries of an ostomy bag, but not a permanent one.

Ruben, third time through chemo because of testicular cancer, his gonads gone, a tube hanging out of his penis, and some bedsores because he had been confined for such a long time to his bed.

Emotionally, spiritually, and physically I can feel his own anguish and torment.

Perhaps these acquaintances and friends I am observing do not have this hollow feeling of an uncontrolled physical deficit or this inability and powerlessness to map out their own future. Perhaps they hang on to a belief that this is what God intends. This is what life is supposed to be about. "Grin and bear it."

"What in the name of any god can I do? I do not want a bodily shattered life in a powered wheelchair ... despite how good and happy the wheelchair company wants you to appear to live: 'You can even see the Grand Canyon in your power chair.'"

I do not want a life like Wilma's, or Ruben's, or Gerry's. Then I recognize what I am feeling: I am terrified.

Yet, as often happens for me—thank whatever gods may be—the rational side creeps into my awareness. I begin to think ... now what? What can I do? And I start to think about searching for alternative solutions.

I left the gathering that afternoon ... and found, when I arrived home, that I was in a safe place for reflection and contemplation. With less terror, and a calming sensitive spirit, I began to ask, "What are my options?"

With journal in hand I wrote: "I guess I could say that "it" is in God's hands. But I don't think God has done a very good job of protecting my friends from the terrifying, empty abyss of "the hellhole of endless paralysis." I can't rely on "it" being in some god's hand."

"What will be will be!" Again, powerlessness. And just waiting to see how it all turns out? No thanks.

"Everything has a reason." Bullshit. That's a New Age emotional dead end. I cannot condone such a shallow interpretation of fate. Never could.

Is my end pre-destined? I never have been a Calvinist—and I'm not going to start now.

I do consider one answer: take charge of my own dying. I have read recently how the professionals—theological gurus, psychiatrists, and attorneys—write and theorize that the idea of controlling your own death goes against God, good mental health, and even the law. But I also know that to be in control of my own death can be objective and rational. I can, I believe, find a way to die – not in chaos, but with dignity.

I have already taken the early precautions. On the advice of my attorney, and with the consent of my family and my primary care doctor, I have written a thorough and detailed advance directive. The family knows that if I have a devastating stroke—one in which I cannot articulate my wishes, and one that will be incurable—then I want to die: no feeding tube, no attempts to keep me alive by all the technology and machines ... no water and no food. Death by fasting.

But the gods wouldn't like that. And when that time comes, I realize that my family could tell the doctors that I wasn't in my right mind when I had made the advance directive decisions. And the doctor or doctors could argue that it was against their moral principles. They would do all that they could to keep me alive. Family, friends, and the church, though progressive in thought, would hide a deep-seated emotional feeling that "he" is going against nature, and therefore against all that is right and human.

There are other options, aren't there?

I had read Derek Humphry's "Final Exit: The Practicalities of Self-Deliverance and Assisted Suicide for the Dying" and was considering those suggestions for a self-inflicted death.

And the latest author who has given me much to think about is a well-known and highly criticized psychiatrist, Thomas S. Szasz.

Szasz wrote:

*"Not long ago the right-thinking person believed that masturbation, oral sex, homosexuality, and other 'unnatural acts' were medical problems whose solution was delegated to doctors. It took us*

*a surprisingly long time to take these behaviors back from physicians, accept them comfortably, and speak about them calmly.*

*Perhaps the time is ripe to rethink our attitude toward suicide and its relation to the medical profession, accept suicide comfortably, and speak about it calmly. To accomplish this, we must demedicalize and destigmatize voluntary death and accept it as a behavior that has always been and will always be a part of the human condition.*

*As individuals, we can choose to die actively or passively, practicing death control or dying of disease or old age. As a society, we can choose to let people die on their own terms or force them to die on terms decreed by the dominant ethic."*

Another thought edged its way into my thinking. I have always been possessed by a strong individualistic and intuitive spirit. I recall reading the poetry of William Ernest Henley when I was in college. Two verses still resonate with my feelings:

> "Out of the night that covers me,
> Black as the pit from pole to pole,
> I thank whatever gods may be
> For my unconquerable soul.
> It matters not how strait the gate,
> How charged with punishments the scroll,
> I am the master of my fate:
> I am the captain of my soul."

Today in my journal I write: "There is a darkness, a fear, about being locked into an unending, terrifying, wordless pathetic stroke. There is the reality I have seen in others of an end-stage downhill slide—where it is obvious that the chemo will not work, a very powerful struggle that grants only a few more months of living, most of it without quality."

I have heard that some argue that living out one's life until the bitter end is what gives life its real value. But, while that does seem to be a factor for some, it is not for all. If the time would come when living seemed to forecast an insurmountable, irretrievable, and very painful death, what would I do?

I would, I decided, make sure that I would try to say my goodbyes by being in touch regularly with family and friends. I would be aware of regrets that I may still harbor – and that I might work through even at this late date in my life.

I would take an unequivocal look at what was being said and written, not only about being in control of my own dying and death, but also what it might mean to place myself in the hands of hospice and other medical professionals who understand fear, pain, and the wishes of the dying person. I know now that my primary care doctor knows that I would like, and I know that he would carry out my wishes.

I do not live in a state that has medical assistance for dying. If I lived in Colorado or any of the dozen states that have laws that allow for medical assistance, that might be my choice.

I will, continue to say to myself, "If the slow and painful dying is about to happen, if there is an inevitable ending of life on this planet, I think I may leave the party early."

## Contributed by Moses Mason –
### Past hospital chaplain and current law student

I've been invited by my friend Ralph to "enter into the dialogue" about death – my own. Death is one of those topics that has been persistent in my mind for the last 35 years or so – and I am 42 years old.

My maternal grandmother died when I was 8. A few years later, her last two siblings died months apart. Their deaths always had my then-mid-30s-year-old mother outwardly talking about her own death throughout my childhood and adolescence. Interesting enough, now that she is months away from turning 70, she has an enthusiasm about life I wished she experienced during my younger years.

My maternal grandmother and her siblings died in hospitals. After being a chaplain in three hospitals, I know for certain I do not want to die in one. The hospital environment is cold. My mother reports that my grandmother felt a sense of loneliness in her final days as she laid in an open hospital ward. Additionally, I do not want my money or the government's money going to make some doctor or hospital executive rich. I want my survivors to take whatever money I have left and live off that money.

At the end of life, hospitals are pointless. After all, the Bible makes clear, death is inevitable and will occur to us all.

I want to live a long life; one that is quality-filled where I maintain some sense of independence and autonomy. I say "some sense" because at some point I will lean on my family and friends to assist me with some basic functions of independent living like driving to get groceries. Houston's highways and streets are increasingly becoming congested. At times – even now when I am fit and healthy -- aggressive drivers make me fearful of getting on the interstate. I do not want to imagine what driving in this city will be like 30-40 years from now.

Like many people, I do not know how my end will come. My late paternal grandmother is my role model for how I want my end to be. As a 93-year-old woman, she lived in her own house with my aunts, uncles, and cousins living nearby. She had been hospitalized about 6 weeks prior to her death and we thought she would die there. Thankfully, she healed enough to be released to her house. One April 2007 evening after eating dinner, she retired to bed. It was there the next morning when my cousin went to see about her, he found that she slept away into the arms of her late husband, two of their children, and her Lord Jesus Christ.

My paternal grandmother had some choice in the timing of her death. In the last ten years of her life, she committed my father to a nursing home after he had a debilitating stroke. More saddening, she buried two of her children. After the second burial, she willed herself to die.

She grieved my uncle's death privately. In her grief, she became forgetful, which was unlike her. Four months prior to her death when we suspected that 2007 would be her last year on earth, my mother, siblings, and I drove to the New Orleans suburbs to say goodbye to her.

When my body gets to the point where I am no longer able to live and function independently, I desire to 'will' myself to die. I hope I will be aware of my impending death as some of my patents were and discontinue any life-sustaining treatments. What does this mean for me? I hope to die in my house or in a hospice facility under comfort measures only. I want enough pain medication to take the edge off any pain I might experience. I want a family member or a friend to be present at my death. That's it.

Why not anything more? Given what I have written about hospitals, finances, and my own need for independence, why not entertain options such as physician-assisted suicide or voluntary assisted euthanasia?

To start with the obvious, I live in Texas and it does not allow for such options. However, if I lived in a state where PAS (Physician Assisted Suicide) or VAE (Active Euthanasia) was allowed, I would seriously look at these options as possibilities for ending my life if I was diagnosed with a terminal illness <u>and</u> death was imminent (6 months – year). Everything Ralph mentioned about living a life with dignity and dying with dignity are ideas that resonate deep within my soul. PAS and VAE would allow me to live and die on *my own* terms. If I chose the day of my death, I would get my affairs in order and say goodbye to my friends and loved ones. Additionally, I would speak my mind and share wisdom on living this life and how I chose to die. Additionally, I would not be a long-term burden to my family. The arguments for PAS and VAE are valid arguments and I wish my state would allow me to have such options.

And then, I would decline these options. Unlike Ralph, I would not "leave the party early" because Texas is where the greatest concentration of my family and friends reside. Furthermore, PAS and VAE would be declined because of my ever-changing Christian faith with some of its constructs built on biblical literalism, a respect for mystery, and some desire to control the narrative of how I lived and died.

The Hebrew Bible book of Ecclesiastes informs much of my current perspective about death and dying. In chapter 7, the wise Teacher says, "For death is the destiny of every man. Why die before your time?" In chapter 11, it is recorded, "No man knows when his hour will come." The Teacher concludes the book by saying, "God will bring every deed into judgement, including every hidden thing, whether it is good or evil." Hebrews 9:27 summarizes it all by saying, "It is appointed unto men once to die, but after this the judgment."

My faith has been and continues to be influenced by the reality of living in the Bible Belt. I was raised in African American Baptist churches. While I no longer attend the conservative churches of my youth, what they instilled in me about life and death persists inside of my soul. Life was given to me by God. It is only God who can take life and breath away. God alone knows when this will happen. Having said such, PAE and VAE are not options available to me because with such options, I believe I am taking this control away from my Maker. This would be sinful in my own eyes and theological constructs.

I cannot always understand the ways of God. This is not to say I have not attempted to figure it out. Oh, I have tried. However, life experiences teach me that this life is one big mystery guided by a series of choices made at crucial decision points. Death is a mystery to me. My paternal grandmother died quickly. My maternal grandmother laid in the hospital for days and was sick for several months prior to her death. I do not know how my own dying process will occur. In my calmer moments, I am ok with this mystery. When I get anxious, I turn to Pierre de Chardin's "Trust in the slow work of God" prayer to ease my concerns and help me to accept mystery. My hope is that if I am given a terminal diagnosis and I am near death, I can remember the opening of his prayer:

*Above all, trust in the slow work of God.*
*We are quite naturally impatient in everything*
*to reach the end without delay.*
*We should like to skip the intermediate stages.*
*We are impatient of being on the way*
*to something unknown, something new.*
*Yet it is the law of all progress that is made*
*by passing through some stages of instability*
*and that may take a very long time.*

If this involves suffering, then I'll accept it. I cannot say I will initially accept it happily and willingly. Knowing myself, I probably will not. I will argue with God and raise my fist to the Divine. I will rail against suffering privately because I would not want any human to tell me to accept suffering because it is the will of God. Knowing myself and how I have operated all these years, at some point I will remember Jesus on the cross. I will remember my mother, grandmothers, mentors, and all my racial ancestors who lived, suffered, and died so I may experience freedom and rights in America. The Christian tradition along with my racial heritage teaches me that suffering can be redemptive if I choose to make it so.

For me, this means there is a lot to learn about myself, others, love, living, and God from the suffering process. My life experiences have affirmed this truth within my soul.

Finally, I would decline PAS and VAE because of the words: "suicide" and "euthanasia." In many African American communities, "suicide" denotes weakness and lack of strength. On a deeper level, suicide is seen as a lack of faith in God. "Euthanasia" is seen as something that some White Americans wish upon the African American community to rid the American continent of its issues around race.

At death, "judgment begins." The Christian tradition is still debating the timing of judgment day, the day when God judges my actions and determines where my soul will eternally reside. The timing of *when* this day will occur is not a concern of mine. However, I am concerned about the narrative that will be constructed by my survivors after my "dust returns to the ground it came from, and the spirit returns to God who gave it" (Ecclesiastes 12:7). This narrative and its construction are judgments of me. I do not want suicide nor euthanasia associated with me or my death.

## Contributed by John Grindler Katonah
Retired Director of Pastoral Care.

The underlying issue is first one of being honest about prioritizing what is each individual's valuing when contemplating their "quality of life". Where is that fine line we each must claim between a purposeful life worth living versus a life devoid of purpose (and maybe without a personalized sense of "dignity")?

Is being of clear mind, thinking, and voicing the proverbial dividing line, or a certain level of mobility, or remaining as an explicitly valued member of a family or community, or a personalized goal desiring to be fulfilled (e.g. attend my daughter's wedding). Where is that fine line we decipher to be true for us existentially?

Related to the above point is a recognition of our experience with suffering (read Eric Cassal, MD on "The Nature of Suffering" found online). Is there something redemptive in our suffering and at what point is our suffering pointless (how we determine this is not always clear because we have no crystal ball to guide us into the future)? But having an understanding for how suffering affects us is vital in sustaining self-compassion for what the sufferer is experiencing.

I recall having multiple hospital visits as a chaplain with a woman in her early thirties who had only within the previous year discovered what was most important in her life: to be a professional softball player. She felt cheated by a new diagnosis of terminal cancer that would prevent her from fulfilling that dream. She began working through deep disappointment and questioning of the meaning of her circumstance during our visits together.

Her suffering was not physical but when confronted by a reality that could not be actualized, she was grief-stricken ... yet how many people live long enough to recognize and seek after what is most precious to them? Her reason to live became clearly defined, so dying was a huge detractor from her life's desire. Purpose then plays a vital role in a person's decisioning to end their life.

I have been with other hospitalized persons who have lost their will to thrive, leading to their medical condition declining to the point of no longer eating or drinking. Eventually this led to death. There is a debate within medical centers these days to change the code and practice of determining a patient's preference for ceasing extraordinary means of maintaining one's life. It is referred to as "do not resuscitate" (commonly referred to among the healthcare team as DNR). What has become our commended reframing of that status is a more positive gesture that also recognizes the natural dying/death process: "allow natural death" (AND). Ultimately, the question comes down to: Does society or the individual have the final say in terminating one's life rather than allowing nature to take its course?

My perspective is that choosing the appropriate length of one's life is an existential discernment process, weighing the benefits versus the liabilities for self, those most affected by the potential loss and its impact on the greater community.

Values, degree of faith in an ultimate source, and past experiences make this process messy and complicated, yet they are an inherent part of what instills human dignity and worth that we all strive for.

## Contributed by Richard Baer
– a new thought from a retired hospice nurse

### "Patient Refusal of Nutrition and Hydration"

Something that is rarely talked about *or* thought about when discussing end-of-life options is refusing nutrition *and* hydration – not simply IVs and tube feedings but all food and fluids. As you know, many – most – of our hospice patients spend their last hours, days, or weeks not able to eat. This does not seem to result in increased discomfort for them, though it may for their loved ones.

My recommendation to many patients who asked me about "self-deliverance" was that they consider fasting from food *and* fluid until they died. No one, of any age, can survive more than 7-10 days – two weeks at the most without food and fluid.

It is (I think!) how I will choose to finish my life when the time comes. Though I'm not at all opposed to active euthanasia, "Patient refusal of nutrition and hydration" has the benefit of not being illegal. Please see the link below for more information. The "Dying Wish" DVD documents the journey of a physician in Boulder who fasted until his death.

"Dying Wish" DVD:
https://www.dyingwishmedia.com/
https://www.youtube.com/watch?v=VNGXbi84U5o

# Ira R. Byock, MD

> Patient Refusal of Nutrition and Hydration: Walking the Ever-Finer Line
>
> American Journal Hospice & Palliative Care, pp. 8-13, March/April 1995.

In the midst of an increasingly heated debate over physician-assisted suicide (PAS) another option available to patients who are determined to end their lives is receiving serious attention, the conscious refusal of nutrition and hydration. Patient refusal of nutrition and hydration (PRNH) is hardly new, indeed, virtually all hospice clinicians remember people who came to a point in their illness when they could be described as having "lost their will to live" and who recognized that continued eating and drinking was having an undesired, life-prolonging effect. In the hospice context, death that follows the decision to refrain from food or drink is not usually considered a suicide, however, by choosing to do so these patients were conscious that their death would likely be hastened.

The general impression among hospice clinicians that starvation and dehydration do not contribute to suffering among the dying and might actually contribute to a comfortable passage from life. In contrast the general impression among the public and non-hospice medical professionals is that starvation and dehydration are terrible ways to die.

Scientific support for either viewpoint has been scanty, yet modern medical practice has reflected an aversion to allowing a person to "starve to death."

Indeed, during the era in which most hospice providers have trained and practiced, a patient unable to eat has been routinely treated with a feeding tube; the option of declining such intervention never having been offered or fully considered. The symbolic importance of offering food and fluids is well-recognized. While it has been utilized by people throughout human history, in public discussion and debates regarding physician-assisted suicide, hospice providers have wisely avoided suggesting PRNH as an alternative. There has been concern that in the political arena such a suggestion might appear as a self-serving way to deny hospice providers' "ultimate responsibility" to the suffering patient.

But the situation may now be changing. Several recent articles are serving to dispel fears of suffering and are making it more acceptable to speak more openly about this inherent ability of patients to influence the timing of their demise. Late in 1993 an article entitled, Patient Refusal of Hydration and Nutrition: An Alternative to Physician-Assisted Suicide or Voluntary Active Euthanasia, by Bernat, et. al. in the Archives of Internal Medicine reviewed the salient clinical literature and discussed the ethical implications of this option. [Bernat] The authors include PRNH within the ethical category of "voluntary passive euthanasia" since it involves not only the refusal of oral food and fluid but the associated refusal of non-oral (enteral or parenteral) alimentation and hydration. They assert that the critical moral and legal distinction to be made regarding a life-ending decision is not whether it involves an act of commission or omission on the part of the physician, but whether or not it constitutes the refusal of a medical therapy by a competent patient. Patient refusal of nutrition and hydration meets this criteria, and thus, can be considered among the commonly accepted practices of patient-initiated refusal (or withdrawal) of mechanical ventilation, renal dialysis, or antibiotic use.

This article is part of a more extensive and thorough article. Go to
https://www.worldrtd.net/patient-refusal-nutrition-and-hydration.

# Katy Butler

*Permission has been given by Katy Butler for the following chapter taken from "The Art of Dying Well."*

## "How to prepare yourself for a good end of life."

By Katy Butler Feb. 17, 2019 Updated: Feb. 17, 2019 3:57 p.m.

Don't wait until you're at death's door to explore your passions, deepen your relationships and find your posse.

My parents lived good lives and expected to die good deaths. They exercised daily, ate plenty of fruits and vegetables, and kept, in their well-organized files, boilerplate advance health directives. But when he was 79, my beloved and seemingly vigorous father came up from his basement study, put on the kettle for tea, and had a devastating stroke. For the next 6½ years, my mother and I watched, heartbroken and largely helpless, as he descended into dementia, near-blindness and misery. To make matters worse, a pacemaker, thoughtlessly inserted two years after his stroke, unnecessarily prolonged his worst years on Earth.

That was a decade ago. Last month I turned 70. The peculiar problems of modern death — often overly medicalized and unnecessarily prolonged — are no longer abstractions to me. Even though I swim daily and take no medications, somewhere beyond the horizon, my death has saddled his horse and is heading my way. I want a better death than many of those I've recently seen.

In this I'm not alone. According to a 2017 Kaiser Foundation study, 7 in 10 Americans hope to die at home. But half die in nursing homes and hospitals, and more than a tenth are cruelly shuttled from one to the other in their final three days. Pain is a major barrier to a peaceful death, and nearly half of dying Americans suffer from uncontrolled pain. Nobody I know hopes to die in the soulless confines of an Intensive Care Unit. But more than a quarter of Medicare members cycle through one in their final month, and a fifth of Americans die in an ICU.

This state-of-affairs has many causes, among them fear, a culture-wide denial of death, ignorance of medicine's limits, and a language barrier between medical staff and ordinary people. "They often feel abandoned at their greatest hour of need," an HMO nurse told me about her many terminally ill patients. "But the oncologists tell us that their patients fire them if they are truthful."

I don't want this to be my story.

In the past three years, I've interviewed hundreds of people who have witnessed good deaths and hard ones, and I consulted top experts in end-of-life medicine. This is what I learned about how to get the best from our imperfect health care system and how to prepare for a good end of life.

Have a vision. Imagine what it would take you to die in peace and work back from there. Whom do you need to thank or forgive? Do you want to have someone reading to you from poetry or the Bible, or massaging your hands with oil, or simply holding them in silence? Talk about this with people you love.

Once you've got the basics clear, expand your horizons. A former forester, suffering from multiple sclerosis, was gurneyed into the woods in Washington state by volunteer firefighters for a last glimpse of his beloved trees. Something like this is possible if you face death while still enjoying life. Appoint someone with people skills and a backbone to speak for you if you can no longer speak for yourself.

Stay in charge. If your doctor isn't curious about what matters to you or won't tell you what's going on in plain English, fire that doctor. That's what Amy Berman did when a prominent oncologist told her to undergo chemotherapy, a mastectomy, radiation and then more chemo to treat her stage-four inflammatory breast cancer.

She settled on another oncologist who asked her, "What do you want to accomplish?" Berman said that she was aiming for a "Niagara Falls trajectory:"

To live as well as possible for as long as possible, followed by a rapid final decline.

Berman, now 59, went on an estrogen suppressing pill. Eight years, later, she's still working, she's climbed the Great Wall of China, and has never been hospitalized. "Most doctors," she says, "focus only on length of life. That's not my only metric."

Know the trajectory of your illness. If you face a frightening diagnosis, ask your doctor to draw a sketch tracking how you might feel and function during your illness and its treatments. A visual will yield far more helpful information than asking exactly how much time you have left.

When you become fragile, consider shifting your emphasis from cure to comfort and find an alternative to the emergency room.

And don't be afraid to explore hospice sooner rather than later. It won't make you die sooner, it's covered by insurance, and you are more likely to die well, with your family supported and your pain under control.

Find your tribe and arrange caregivers. Dying at home is labor-intensive. Hospices provide home visits from nurses and other professionals, but your friends, relatives and hired aides will be the ones who empty bedpans and provide hands-on care. You don't have to be rich, or a saint, to handle this well.

You do need one fiercely committed person to act as a central tent pole and as many part-timers as you can marshal. People who die comfortable, well-supported deaths at home tend to have one of three things going for them: money, a rich social network of neighbors or friends, or a good government program (like PACE, the federal Program of All-Inclusive Care for the Elderly).

Don't wait until you're at death's door to explore your passions, deepen your relationships and find your posse. Do favors for your neighbors and mentor younger people. It doesn't matter if you find your allies among fellow quilters, bridge-players, tai chi practitioners, or in the Christian Motorcyclists Association. You just need to share an activity face-to-face.

Take command of the space. No matter where death occurs, you can bring calm and meaning to the room. Don't be afraid to rearrange the physical environment. Weddings have been held in ICUs so that a dying mother could witness the ceremony. In a hospital or nursing home, ask for a private room, get televisions and telemetry turned off, and stop the taking of vital signs.

Clean house: Hospice nurses often list five emotional tasks for the end of life: thank you, I love you, please forgive me, I forgive you, and goodbye. Do not underestimate the power of your emotional legacy, expressed in even a small, last-minute exchange. Kathy Duby of Mill Valley was raised on the East

Coast by a violent alcoholic mother. She had no memory of ever hearing, "I love you."

When Duby was in her 40s, her mother lay dying of breast cancer in a hospital in Boston. Over the phone, she told Duby, "Don't come, I don't want to see you." Duby got on a plane anyway.

She walked into the hospital room to see a tiny figure curled up in bed — shrunken, yellow, bald, bronzed by jaundice, as Duby later wrote in a poem. Duby's mother said aloud, "I love you and I'm sorry."

Duby replied, "I love you and I'm sorry."

"Those few moments," Duby said, "Cleared up a lifetime of misunderstanding each other."

Think of death as a rite of passage. In the days before effective medicine, our ancestors were guided by books and customs that framed dying as a spiritual ordeal rather than a medical event. Without abandoning the best of what modern medicine has to offer, return to that spirit.

Over the years, I've learned one thing: Those who contemplate their aging, vulnerability and mortality often live better lives and experience better deaths than those who don't. They enroll in hospice earlier, and often feel and function better — and sometimes even live longer — than those who pursue maximum treatment.

We influence our lives, but we don't control them, and the same goes for how they end. No matter how bravely you adapt to loss and how cannily you navigate our fragmented health system, dying will still represent the ultimate loss of control.

But you don't have to be a passive victim. You retain moral agency. You can keep shaping your life all the way to its end — as long as you seize the power to imagine, to arrange support and to plan.

# Statement from Anton van Niekerk

*I am using the following quote from Anton van Niekerk as a narrative that names the issues that define what is involved in 'medically assisted dying."*

*Note Niekerk's use of the word 'euthanasia' – and "medically assisted suicide." Current language would be "medically assisted dying".*

*The following is lengthy but very relevant. I am in agreement with Niekerk. I hope for and wish for an option other than an insurmountable, irretrievable, and very painful death.*

*I will, in finding clarity, define more specifically my advanced standing goals. And I will share those with my children, Joel and Jill, and with partner Keo.*

**Anton van Niekerk:** Distinguished Professor of Philosophy and Director: Centre for Applied Ethics, Stellenbosch University. Stellenbosch University provides funding as a partner of The Conversation AFRICA.

*Republish our articles for free, online or in print, under Creative Commons license.*

"Desmond Tutu said on his 85th birthday early in October 2016 that he wanted the right to end his life through (medically) assisted dying.

Euthanasia represents one of the oldest issues in medical ethics. It is forbidden in the original Hippocratic Oath, and has consistently been opposed by most religious traditions since antiquity – other than, incidentally, abortion, which has only been formally banned by the Catholic Church since the middle of the 19th century.

Euthanasia is a wide topic with many dimensions. I will limit myself in this article to the issue of **"assisted death"**, which seems to me to be one of the most pressing issues of our time.

Desmond Tutu, emeritus archbishop of Cape Town, raised it again on his 85th birthday in an article in the Washington Post. He wrote: *"I have prepared for my death and have made it clear that I do not wish to be kept alive at all costs. I hope I am treated with compassion and allowed to pass onto the next phase of life's journey in the manner of my choice."*

Assisted dying can take the form of physician assisted suicide (PAS). Here a suffering and terminal patient is assisted by a physician to gain access to a lethal substance which the patient himself or herself takes or administers. If incapable of doing so, the physician – on request of the patient – administers the lethal substance which terminates the patient's life.

(Currently State laws usually require the patient to be conscious and able to take the pill.)

The latter procedure is also referred to as "voluntary active euthanasia" (VAE). I will not deal with the issue of involuntary euthanasia –where the suffering patient's life is terminated without their explicit consent -– a procedure which, to my mind, is ethically much more problematic.

**Passive form of euthanasia**

The term "voluntary active euthanasia" suggests that there also is a passive form of euthanasia. It is passive in the sense that nothing is "actively" done to kill the patient, but that nothing is done to deter the process of dying either. The termination of life-support which is clearly futile is permitted.

However, the moral significance of the distinction between "active" and "passive" euthanasia is increasingly questioned by ethicists. The reason simply is the credibility of arguing that administering a lethal agent is "active," but terminating life support (for example switching off a ventilator) is "passive". Both clearly are observable and describable actions, and both are the direct causes of the patient's death.

There are a number of reasons for the opposition to physician assisted suicide or voluntary active euthanasia. The value bestowed on human life in all religious traditions and almost all cultures, such as the prohibition on murder, is so pervasive that it is an element of common, and not statutory, law.

Objections from the medical profession to being seen or utilized as "killers" rather than saviors of human life, as well as the sometimes well-founded fear of the possible abuse of physician assisted suicide or voluntary active euthanasia, is a further reason. The main victims of such possible abuse could well be the most vulnerable and indigent members of society: the poor, the disabled and the like. Those who cannot pay for prolonged accommodation in expensive health care facilities and intensive care units.

**Death with dignity**

*In support of physician assisted suicide or voluntary active euthanasia, the argument is often made that, as people have the right to live with dignity, they also have the right to die with dignity. Some medical conditions are simply so painful and unnecessarily prolonged that the capability of the medical profession to alleviate suffering by means of palliative care is surpassed.*

Intractable terminal suffering robs the victims of most of their dignity. In addition, medical science and practice is currently capable of an unprecedented prolongation of human life. It can be a prolongation that too often results in a concomitant prolongation of unnecessary and pointless suffering.

Enormous pressure is placed upon both families and the health care system to spend time and very costly resources on patients that have little or no chance of recovery and are irrevocably destined to die. It is, so the argument goes, not inhumane or irreverent to assist such patients – particularly if they clearly and repeatedly so request – to bring their lives to an end.

I am personally much more in favor of the pro-PAS and pro-VAE positions, although the arguments against do raise issues that need to be addressed. Most of those issues (for example the danger of the exploitation of vulnerable patients) I believe, can be satisfactorily dealt with by regulation.

**Argument in favor of assisted suicide**
*(language is now medically assisted dying)*

The most compelling argument in favor of physician assisted (dying) or voluntary active euthanasia is the argument in support of committing suicide in a democracy. The right to commit suicide is, as far as I am concerned, simply one of the prices we have to be willing to pay as citizens of a democracy.

We do not have the right, and we play no discernible role, in coming into existence. But we do have the right to decide how long we remain in existence. The fact that we have the right to suicide, does not mean that it is always (morally) right to execute that right.

It is hard to deny the right of an 85-year-old with terminal cancer of the pancreas and almost no family and friends left, to commit suicide or ask for assisted death. In this case, he or she both has the right, and will be in the right if exercising that right.

Compare that with the situation of a 40-year-old man, a husband and father of three young children, who has embezzled company funds and now has to face the music in court. He, also, has the right to commit suicide. However, I would argue, it would not be morally right for him to do so, given the dire consequences for his family. To have a right, does not imply that it is always right to execute that right.

My argument in favor of physician assisted suicide or voluntary active euthanasia is thus grounded in the right to suicide, which I think is fundamental to a democracy.

Take the case of a competent person who is terminally ill, who will die within the next six months and has no prospect of relief or cure. This person suffers intolerably and/or intractably, often because of an irreversible dependence on life-support. This patient repeatedly, say at least twice a week, requests that his/her life be terminated. I am convinced that to perform physician assisted suicide or voluntary active euthanasia in this situation is not only the humane and respectful, but the morally justified way to go.

The primary task of the medical profession is not to prolong life or to promote health, but to relieve suffering. We have a right to die with dignity, and the medical profession has a duty to assist in that regard."

# National Hospice and Palliative Care Organization (NHPCO)

Contributed by Sydney Shepherd, *Policy and Advocacy Specialist*

Hospice Action Network /National Hospice and Palliative Care Organization

# Statement on Legally Accelerated Death

**POSITION**

National Hospice and Palliative Care Organization (NHPCO) supports individuals' rights to exercise autonomy as is legal in their communities and seeks to provide assistance to member organizations in communities where legally accelerated death (LAD) is an option. Nevertheless, NHPCO opposes LAD as a societal option to alleviate suffering.

**RATIONALE**

Known as physician assisted suicide (PAS), physician aid in dying (PAD), medical aid in dying (MAID), and other terms, LAD is both controversial and increasingly available to terminally ill individuals in the United States. However, as palliative care "intends to neither hasten nor postpone death," [1] LAD is not a palliative intervention. In light of the underuse of hospice and palliative care to alleviate suffering, lack of comprehensive health care for persons with serious illness, lack of research about the outcomes of LAD, concerns of disability rights advocates regarding protections from coercion, longstanding racial bias in medicine, disparities in health and medical care, and lack of protections to ensure voluntary participation, NHPCO opposes LAD as a societal option.

**NHPCO COMMITMENT of SUPPORT**

Committed to "a world where individuals and families facing serious illness, death, and grief will experience the best that humankind can offer," (2) NHPCO calls on member organizations and others to help "lead and mobilize social change for improved care at the end of life" (3) by advocating for early inclusion of, and improved access to, palliative and hospice care in the management of serious illness.

NHPCO earnestly supports the timely provision of palliative and hospice care to all patients, including those choosing LAD. Sources of actual and potential suffering should be assessed and specific interventions offered to prevent and/or reduce suffering experienced by patients, families, and other caregivers. NHPCO commits to help hospice and palliative care organizations through dissemination of best clinical and regulatory practices and identification of exemplar organizational policies and guidelines pertinent to LAD.

Adopted: November 4, 2018 Expires: (November 2023)

1 World Health Organization. "WHO Definition of Palliative Care." http://www.who.int/cancer/palliative/definition/en/. Accessed May 14, 2018.

2 NHPCO Vision. NHPCO. https://www.nhpco.org/nhpco-0. Accessed May 14, 2018.

3 NHPCO Mission. NHPCO. https://www.nhpco.org/nhpco-. Accessed May 14, 2018.bid.

# Part III

### The Right to Die – my personal view

I am not clear where the issue of 'the right to die' first surfaced in my life. Nevertheless, in recent years the personal *right* to die has become imperative, a thoughtful journey.

The 'right to die' phrase means - among other things- taking on the responsibility to consider options for how I will die.

How could it be otherwise? If I do not, personally, have the 'right to die', then it would seem that someone else or a god somewhere has the distinctive and perhaps obligation to have something to do with my death.

Most people would say it is …. God …. or perhaps Fate. Many, in other words, without resistance, simply turn their dying over to the gods, or fates, or circumstances. No questions, no exploration.

Most resist taking on the sometimes very difficult ethic of …. "I have a right to say something or act on my own behalf when it comes to dying."

*Why difficult?*

Because such an ethic or thought has not been taught. In the past, yes, but seldom in the curriculum of churches or synagogues, or in high schools or colleges or universities.

In college, my major was General Psychology, and in graduate school – Bethany Theological Seminary - very little - perhaps nothing – was focused on 'the right to die.'

In one college course "World's Great Religions" we read a few of the ancient philosophers, but I do not recall in that course that we intentionally philosophized on the author's view of death and dying. It was, of course, on how to live with good intent and integrity. Life with dignity.

Seldom, as I recall, did we, in class, explore the ethical, religious, philosophical roots of the right to die. In fact, in hospice work we assumed that we lived in the ethical dimension of 'we have the right to neither extend the life of the patient, nor hurry the death.'

Now, after years of working and relating to other staff and to patients in hospice or in ministry, I find it worthy to consider the ethical, legal and religious dynamics of dying with dignity.

There is another important dimension to my choosing how I wish to approach my death.

Earlier, John Katonah wrote: "My perspective is that choosing the appropriate length of one's life is an existential discernment process, weighing the benefits versus the liabilities for myself, those most affected by the potential loss, and its impact on the greater community."

*How does how I die effect my family?*

When I choose a natural path of illness and dying, that is, for instance;

a) Treatment until the treatment no longer works, then palliative care – with or without – hospice, and then death.

b) Or I choose to be deliberate in closing out my life earlier by not taking as many possible treatments, or by going as early as possible into hospice care, or choosing to stop both food and water, i.e. – if I recognize that there are deliberate and specific options ... does that have a negative or positive effect on my loved ones? Do they see courage in either choice?

I downloaded and carefully considered the questions and worksheets of "My End of Life Decisions Guide Toolkit."

The following relates some of my thoughts and wishes.

**What are my values and what is important to me when I am dying?**

I wish to participate in making my own decisions about healthcare and treatment. And *always* want to know the truth about my condition, treatment options, and the chance of success of the treatment.

I choose hospice support, alertness (morphine, but not making me unaware), family and friends present and supportive, anointing with Pastor Katie and family/friends present , comfort and little pain, that others understand and accept my choices for my dying process, and that there will be little or no attempt to extend my life.

I wish for no life-sustaining measures in cases of terminal illness, permanent coma, and dementia. In the event of irreversible chronic illness – if life-sustaining measures allows some quality of life and awareness, then some measures are okay. When the chronic illness becomes very painful or leads into unconsciousness or my inability to make final decisions, then no more life-sustaining measures.

When disease is terminal and I have made the request of no CPR then I want no permanent mechanical breathing, no CPR, no artificial nutrition (feeding tube), limited hydration or perhaps no hydration (I will make that choice at the time), and no hospital intensive care.

I am okay with pain-relief medication, okay with antibiotics if for pain relief, okay with chemo or radiation if still in stage one or two but not beyond, okay with surgery if I am conscious and able to make the choice.

If I am physically and permanently incapacitated, and have terminal illness, I would likely make decisions for finality as soon as possible.

If it was clear that I was moving toward dementia/Alzheimer's I would make decisions for finality. Difficult problem would be that I might not be physically incapacitated.

If I was alone and I would have to go into nursing care, I would choose to make finality decisions. I would probably choose to stop nutrition and hydration.

I am willing to be placed in a nursing home or care facility, but only if I was in hospice care. I would prefer to be in hospice care in my home. Hospitalization would be my second choice – in hospice care. A nursing home is the last choice. Even then, in hospice care.

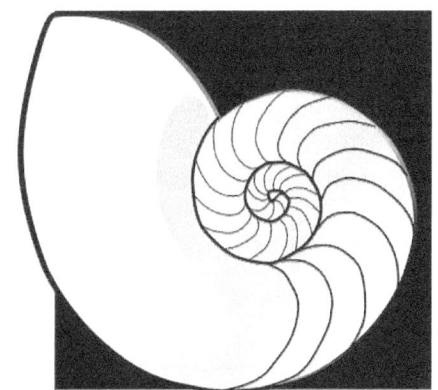

# The Chambered Nautilus

An image that has been of great importance to me is the Chambered Nautilus. I wrote in my book "Into the Next Chamber" the following.

The Introduction read:

"Recently, because of a life-threatening disease and my advancing age, the image of the Chambered Nautilus, poem and shell, has had a particular and powerful significance.

The living Nautilus is fascinating! This sea creature repeatedly continues in its life's journey by moving into a new and larger chamber. Oliver Wendell Holmes writes of the Nautilus: "He left the past year's dwelling for the new . . . Stretched in his last-found home and knew the old no more." Holmes continues: "Build thee more stately mansions, O my soul, As the swift seasons roll, Leave thy low-vaulted past."

What a striking and challenging metaphor! In each moment, in each day and year of our lives, *we build a new chamber*. We initiate the next step of our journey by courageously moving into that new, unknown promise.

Our life existence and experience is in moving ahead, not in staying behind. If we do not build a new chamber and try to stay in the old, we are fatally locked into that "secure cocoon" and eventually are so chained and shackled that we are eventually squeezed to death by the confines of the past. Perhaps not a bodily death, but certainly a spiritual death.

On its journey into the next chamber the Nautilus does so in order to survive.

For any of us, moving into that new chamber is a matter of survival --- and it is risky. We leave our security behind. We leave what is safe and familiar.
We may not live up to the spirit of the ancient Nautilus, but the challenge is there: lead off into a new and yet unexplored space. Risk the unknown future. An understanding and appreciation of the Chambered Nautilus is, for me, a way to perceive and accept the dignity of living and of dying. It is a spiritual and human acknowledgement.

"Life is meant to be lived from a Center, a divine Center...Life from the Center is a life of unhurried peace and power. It is simple. It is serene. It is amazing. It is triumphant. It is radiant. It takes no time, but it occupies all our time. And it makes our life programs new and overcoming. We need not get frantic. He is at the helm. And when our little day is done, we lie down quietly in peace, for all is well."
— Thomas R. Kelly, <u>A Testament of Devotion</u>

# Religion and Spirituality

*Following is an extended quote from the national site of Death with Dignity.*

Though extensive, the noting of the many attitudes of the various world's religions, basically underscores that *religion has had a major role in determining the attitudes of our human culture.*

Fortunately, some religious and faith-based groups have had a more enlightened perspective. For some, <u>it is imperative that a terminally ill patient be allowed to hasten an inevitable and unavoidable death.</u>

While many faith traditions adhere to ancient traditions and understandings of physical life's final journey, modern medical technology has opened the door for faith leaders to actively reconsider some beliefs.

Death with Dignity laws offer dying individuals an opportunity to ponder an important final life question: "What is the meaning of my life?"

For many this is a profoundly spiritual question to which answers come not when an individual is consumed by a flurry of doctor's appointments, treatments or tests, but in the comfort of solitude, when the individual feels at peace.

As the leading edge of public policy working to ensure the rights of patients on this important final journey, Death with Dignity is not only a legal issue, but a cultural and spiritual issue as well. Some faith traditions have embraced Death with Dignity as an ultimate act of compassion, and others reject it is as morally bankrupt practice.

*Below are summaries of viewpoints of differing faith traditions on Death with Dignity.* There is as much diversity among different faith traditions as there is between them. This research is the work of Compassion and Choices.

**Note:** *Pro-choice statements have been made by the United Church of Christ, and the Methodist Church on the US West Coast.*

*The Episcopalian (Anglican), Unitarian Universalist, Methodist, Presbyterian and Quaker movements are among the most liberal, allowing at least individual decision-making in cases of hastened death.*

*Added into the following list is the Church of the Brethren, similar in history to Mennonite and Quaker. Church of the Brethren is not a part of the original list.*

### *Anglican*

*Rowan Williams, the Anglican Archbishop of Canterbury, has stated that, although "there is a very strong compassionate case" for physician-assisted dying, the Anglican church remains opposed to the practice.*

### *Baptist*

*The American Baptists Churches and Southern Baptist Convention differ in their statements regarding assisted dying. The American Baptists have adopted the policy "to advocate within the medical community for increased emphasis on the caring goals of medicine which preserve the dignity and minimize the suffering of the individual and respect personal choice for end of life care." The Southern Baptists state this end-of-life option violates the sanctity of human life.*

### *Buddhist*

*The teachings of the Buddha don't explicitly deal with aid in dying, but the Buddha himself showed tolerance of suicide by monks in two cases. Buddhists are not unanimous in their view of physician-assisted dying. The Japanese Buddhist tradition includes many stories of suicide by monks; suicide was used as a political weapon by Buddhist monks during the Vietnam war. In Buddhism, the way life ends has a profound impact on the way the new, reincarnated life will begin. So a person's state of mind at the time of death is important: their thoughts should be selfless and enlightened, free of anger, hate or fear. This suggests that suicide is only appropriate for people who have achieved enlightenment and that the rest of us should avoid it.*

**(Additional note from Buddhist Richard Baer)**

"The notion that one's mind should be at peace at the moment of death is, indeed, very important in the Buddhist tradition. This is one of the reasons that I have been a DNR patient for 20 years, despite my general good health. I do not want my last moments in this *incarnation to be at the end of defibrillator paddles. I have, during several surgeries, revoked my DNR during the surgery and said that they could perform CPR for 3 minutes MAXIMUM if I arrested.*

*Regarding suicide, though it is officially considered not a good thing to do, most Western Buddhists I know generally feel positive about "pro-choice" in matters of abortion rights and the right to die.*

*I'm aware of one instance where the American student of a Thai Buddhist monk had a very intractably painful condition that was not terminal. He said that she should not take her own life but supported her decision to fast until her death (a process that takes 7-10 days)."*

**Roman Catholic**

The official position of the Roman Catholic Church is strict: the killing of a human being, even by an act of omission to eliminate suffering, violates divine law and offends the *dignity of the human person. However, many Catholics—particularly in the United States—cite various quotations by Pope Benedict XVI as a source for continued disagreement and controversy regarding these controversial issues. To compound confusion, physician-assisted dying is frequently and erroneously considered euthanasia:*

- *"Freedom to kill is not a true freedom but a tyranny that reduces the human being into slavery."*
- *"Scripture, in fact, clearly excludes every form of the kind of self-determination of human existence that is presupposed in the theory and practice of euthanasia."*
- *"Not all moral issues have the same moral weight as abortion and euthanasia. For example, if a Catholic were to be at odds with the Holy Father on the application of capital punishment or on the decision to wage war, he would not for that reason be considered unworthy to present himself to receive Holy Communion."*

- *"While the Church exhorts civil authorities to seek peace, not war, and to exercise discretion and mercy in imposing punishment on criminals, it may still be permissible to take up arms to repel an aggressor or to have recourse to capital punishment. There may be a legitimate diversity of opinion even among Catholics about waging war and applying the death penalty, but not however with regard to abortion and euthanasia."*

*Pope Francis, despite being considered more liberal than past popes, has continued statements against physician-hastened death, stating that the practice is "false compassion" and a result of our "throwaway culture" that devalues and dehumanizes the sick. Catholic organizations are often in the lead in organizing against Death with Dignity laws or ballot initiatives.*

### Christian Reformed (Church in North America)

*In 1971 a Synod adopted a resolution which stated: "that synod, mindful of the Sixth*

*Commandment, condemn the wanton or arbitrary destruction of any human being at any state of its development from the point of conception to the point of death."*

### Christian Scientist

*The Church's experience with healing indicates hastened dying is not a genuine expression of faith and is a denial of God's presence and power.*

### Church of the Brethren

*For a full statement go to:*
[http://www.brethren.org/ac/statements/1996endoflife.html](http://www.brethren.org/ac/statements/1996endoflife.html)

a) **Reverence for Life**. How do we live life to its fullest as death approaches?

*Every life is important and precious in the sight of God, as affirmed by numerous Annual Conference statements. The active and intentional taking of life, including assisted suicide, is unacceptable. Also unacceptable, however, is allowing human pain and suffering to go unrelieved, or prolonging the dying process with extraordinary medical interventions. When death approaches, relief of pain and suffering is a higher value than simply prolonging life. Every available resource for relief, such as prayer, meditation, pain management techniques, pain clinics, hospice, and medication should be considered. The spiritual, emotional, relational, and physical nurture offered in love and compassion by family, friends, congregations, and professional caregivers, assists people to die with dignity and respect.*

> **b) Mutual Respect.** *How do we respect the wishes, values, and decisions of people who are dying or bereaved?*

*There is no one right way to die or to grieve. Those who seek to be caring will not force their own views on those who are suffering, dying, or grieving but will remember that the ministry of presence is most important, and that listening is more helpful than giving advice. The wishes and values of those who are dying and grieving, including their decisions about medical care or other approaches to health care, are to be valued and respected.*

**Disciples of Christ**
*The customary reasons for assisted dying, suffering and irreversible conditions, are nullified by the biblical witness to meaningful suffering and to possible healing.*

**Eastern Orthodox**
*Physician assisted dying is morally and theologically impermissible because of God's sovereignty and the sanctity of human life. "Death is seen as evil in itself, and symbolic of all those forces which oppose God-given life and its fulfillment. Salvation and redemption are normally understood in Eastern Christianity in terms of sharing in Jesus Christ's victory over death, sin and evil through His crucifixion and His resurrection. The Orthodox Church has a very strong pro-life stand which in part*

*expresses itself in opposition to doctrinaire advocacy of euthanasia."*

### Episcopal

*Some Episcopalians believe it is morally wrong to take human life with medication to relieve suffering caused by incurable illness. Others approve of assisted dying in rare cases.*

### Evangelical

*While the National Association of Evangelicals (NAE) opposes physician-assisted dying, the NAE "believes that in cases where patients are terminally ill, death appears imminent and treatment offers no medical hope for a cure, it is morally appropriate to request the withdrawal of life-support systems, allowing natural death to occur. In such cases, every effort should be made to keep the patient free of pain and suffering, with emotional and spiritual support being provided until the patient dies."*

### Evangelical Lutheran

*A 1992 statement on end-of-life matters from the Evangelical Lutheran Church of America Council supports physician-assisted death: "Health care professionals are not required to use all available medical treatment in all circumstances. Medical treatment may be limited in some instances, and death allowed to occur." They oppose euthanasia because "deliberately destroying life created in the image of God is contrary to our Christian conscience." However, they do acknowledge that physicians "struggle to choose the lesser evil" in some situations, e.g. when pain is so severe "that life is indistinguishable from torture." Surprisingly, even though Death with Dignity is a hotly debated topic, they do not comment on it.*

### Hindu

*There are several Hindu points of view on physician aid in dying. Most Hindus would say that a doctor should not accept a patient's request for death since this will cause the soul and body to be separated at an unnatural time. The result will damage the karma of both doctor and patient. Other Hindus believe that physician-hastened dying cannot be allowed because it breaches the teaching of ahimsa (doing no harm). However, some Hindus say that by helping to end a painful life a person is performing a good deed and fulfilling their moral obligations.*

## Jainism

*Jains believe that the soul has always been here and cannot be destroyed and that through the process of death, one transitions to a new body. The Jain tradition shows how we can move without attachment into death rather than clinging to life. In their acceptance of the inevitable, Jains set an example that death is not an evil but an opportunity to reflect on a life well-lived and look forward to what lies ahead. Fasting to death is a key religious observance for Janists; those at the end of life can choose to embrace a final fast transition from one body to another.*

***Jehovah's Witness***
*Physician assisted death violates the sanctity of life and Christian conscience.*

***Judaism***
*The Union of Orthodox Jewish Congregations has been heavily involved in efforts, in both Congress and the courts, to restrict physician assisted death. In 2000, Rabbi J. David Bleich, Jewish Law Professor at Yeshiva University's rabbinical seminary and Law Professor at Yeshiva's Cardozo Law School, stated that "Judaism places the highest importance on palliation of pain, particularly in the case of terminal patients," and that "Judaism teaches that suicide is an offense against the Deity who is the Author of life." Conservative and Reform leaders have called for increased discussion of end-of-life issues, and have not issued official positions on assisted dying.*

***Lutheran Church – Missouri Synod***
*"Advocates of euthanasia, as well as of assisted suicide, have sought to justify the taking of*

*human life on moral grounds by describing it as a truly compassionate act aimed at the relief of human suffering. In light of what the Scriptures say about the kind of care God wills that we provide to those who suffer and are facing death, we reject such claims as neither compassionate nor caring. Christians aim always to care, never to kill."*

**Mennonite**

*The Mennonite denomination is a decentralized faith group in which individual conferences make their own statements on social issues. The Conference of Mennonites in Canada issued a statement on the matter in 1995: they believe that pain, isolation and fear are the main factors that drive dying persons to consider suicide and that the state should not facilitate suicide, but rather control physical and emotional pain and support the dying within a caring community setting.*

***Methodist***

*Methodists generally accept the individual's freedom of conscience to determine the means and timing of death. Some regional conferences have endorsed the legalization of medical aid in dying.*

***Mormon***

*Euthanasia is condemned. Anyone who takes part in euthanasia, including assisted suicide, is regarded as having violated the commandments of God. However, the Church recognizes that when a person is in the final stages of terminal illness there may be difficult decisions to be taken. The Church states that, "When dying becomes inevitable, death should be looked upon as a blessing and a purposeful part of an eternal existence. Members should not feel obligated to extend mortal life by means that are unreasonable."*

***Muslim***

*Muslims are against physician-assisted dying. They believe that all human life is sacred because it is given by Allah, and that Allah chooses how long each person will live. Human beings should not interfere in this. This end-of-life option is, therefore, forbidden. Physicians must not take active measures to terminate a patient's life. The Qur'an states: "Take not life which Allah made sacred otherwise than in the course of justice"*

*An essay on the web page of the Islamic Center of Southern California states that "Since we did not create ourselves, we do not own our bodies…Attempting to kill oneself is a crime in Islam as well as a grave sin. The Qur'an says: 'Do not kill (or destroy) yourselves, for verily Allah has been to you most Merciful.' (Quran 4:29) The concept of a life not worthy of living does not exist in Islam."*

### **Presbyterian**
*A 1988 Presbyterian Church position paper on "heroic measures" states that, "Euthanasia, or 'mercy-killing' of a patient by a physician or by anyone else, including the patient himself*

*(suicide) is murder. To withhold or to withdraw medical treatment, as is being discussed here, does not constitute euthanasia and should not be placed into the same category with it."* However, Presbyterians are devoting further study and discussion to the specific issue of physician-assisted dying.

### Russian Orthodox
*The practice of painlessly putting to death people suffering from incurable diseases, contradicts Christian morals, believes official spokesman for the Moscow Patriarchate Father Vsevolod Chaplin.*

### Sikh
*The Sikhs rejected suicide (and by extension, euthanasia) as an interference in God's plan. Suffering, they said, was part of the operation of karma, and human beings should not only accept it without complaint but act so as to make the best of the situation that karma has given them. This is not absolute. Sikhism believes that life is a gift from God, but it also*

*teaches that we have a duty to use life in a responsible way. Therefore, Sikhs contemplating hastening their own or another person's death should look at the whole picture and make appropriate distinctions between ending life and not artificially prolonging a terminal state.*

### Spiritualist

*Through their Life and Death with Dignity policy, National Spiritualist Association of Churches "affirms the right of each individual to determine for self, or through a guardian the extent through which the medical community or family may interfere with the treatment of a terminal, or irreversible condition, by the use of Living Wills, Advanced Directive and Durable Power of Attorneys, available in all states in various form. We as Spiritualists are bound to follow the law. If we, as individuals, would have the current laws changed or extended beyond their present scope, it is our individual right to work for this through the proper channels."*

### *Synod of the Great Lakes – Reformed Church in America*

*"When we consider how Christian convictions influence a choice for assisted suicide, the primary concern is not to protect or deny peoples' rights, but to explain why Christians, given their convictions, are apt to see something as right or wrong. On the whole, Christians value the individual liberty that allows them to act on the basis of their distinctive moral commitments. However, a shared Christian commitment does not seem to be consistent with a choice to take one's own life, even under conditions of extreme suffering."*

### *Unitarian Universalist*

*Unitarian Universalists support Death with Dignity. In its 1988 General Resolution, the Unitarian Universalist Association resolved to advocate for "the right to self-determination in dying" and to "support legislation that will create legal protection for the right to die with dignity, in accordance with one's own choice."*

### United Church of Christ

*The UCC generally affirms individual freedom and responsibility, including the right to choose in regards to reproductive rights, and has a history of encouraging inclusive discussion about all aspects of death and dying.*

*At its 9th General Synod in 1973, the UCC adopted The Rights and Responsibilities of Christians Regarding Human Death, which, inter alia, "affirms the right to die and execution of living wills; supports the right to die with dignity through termination of extraordinary measures to keep a terminally ill, unconscious patient alive..." However, the Synod "did not address the question of euthanasia at a conscious patient's request."*

*At its 26th General Synod, in 2008, the resolution "Legalization of Physician Aid in Dying" was adopted that "called on the church to study a proposal favoring legalization" of "physician aid in dying." The working group established to that end failed to find consensus on the matter. At the 27th General Synod, UCC's*

*Executive Council sent a draft resolution "In Support of Physician Assistance in Dying" back to the working group for further study. Many UCC clergy have been supportive of right-to-die legislation, and the UCC continues to encourage open, inclusive conversations about all aspects of death and dying.*

# Part IV

# Conclusions

## Wherever You Go

**With permission from:**

© 1972 The Benedictine Foundation of the State of Vermont

1. Wherever you go I shall go.
Wherever you live so shall I live.
Your people will be my people,
and your God will be my God too.

Recite:

I want to say something to all of you
who have become a part
of the fabric of my life.

The color and texture
which you have brought into my being
have become a song,
and I want to sing it forever.

There is an energy in us
which makes things happen
when the paths of other persons
touch ours
and we have to be there
and let it happen.

When the time
of our particular sunset comes
our thing, our accomplishment,
won't really matter a great deal.

But the clarity and care
with which we have loved others
will speak with vitality
of the great gift of life
we have been for each other.

2. Wherever you die, I shall die,
and there shall I be buried beside you.
We will be together forever,
and our love will be the gift of our life.

Contributed by Richard Baer

# Louis Shattuck Baer, MD

My Uncle Louis was a person of dignity and integrity. He was an internist beginning in 1939, served in the navy during WWII and lived with his wife, Eve, and three children in the Bay area (Burlingame, CA). In 1953 he contracted polio and lost control of his intercostal muscles which impacted his breathing for the rest of his life. Once he recovered, he resumed practicing medicine, retiring at about age 75.

He spent the last decade of his practice sleeping in a hospital bed with the head of the bed elevated. He continued making house calls until he retired. Uncle Louis felt very strongly about a patient's right to control his/her care. He wrote a book in the late 60s (I think) called, "Let the Patient Decide: A Doctor's Advice to Older People", which included the then outrageous suggestion that a physician NOT treat infections in dementia patients, rather letting them die of the infection and treating them for comfort only.

Beginning in the 1950s, after his polio, my uncle talked about ending his own life if his quality of life had declined. In January of 1988 my uncle had been experiencing intermittent TIAs but more urgently, my Aunt Eve had been diagnosed with pancreatic cancer. They decided to end their lives together. They rented a small apartment and, on the night of

January 21, 1988 went there with their old dog and all three took (the dog was given) a lethal overdose of barbiturates for which my uncle had written a prescription. He had letters that were to be delivered to his children later at which time their bodies were found. My aunt's body was still alive, though she died a few hours later.

The newspaper (San Jose Mercury) wrote about their deaths saying, "At the end of hope, couple die together." (see pdf) but I don't think they were at the end of hope nor were they depressed.

This is the last journal entry my uncle wrote...

January 21, 1988

Thoughts on the last night of my life:

Eve and I feel completely tranquil, content, relaxed and fulfilled.

We believe that together we have experienced the highest type of love, and the greatest intellectual and spiritual joys it is given to man to feel.

We have suffered no more than our allotted share of human suffering, misfortune and sorrow.

We have been greatly enriched by our children, grandchildren and friends.

We leave you with only praise for our Maker and gratitude for the instant of eternity we have shared with each other.

I remain an optimist to the last.

What is good for mankind will survive
 and what is maleficent will ultimately perish.

LSB (Louis Shattuck Baer)

## I'll Be on My Way
### by Ralph McFadden

Regardless of my best efforts to be rational and cogent, it sometimes becomes apparent that heartfelt emotions are exactly that—felt in the heart. I may try to objectify my beliefs, but such a thought process does not begin to explain the whole of one's life.

So it is with a song written by Shawn Kirchner. Shawn is an exceptional writer and composer. On the last cut of his album, "Meet Me on the Mountain," for me, despite my disclaimer of needing no assurance about an afterlife, he catches the delightful situation of being caught up in and wondering about being "glory bound."

In other words, I find this verse and song exhilarating. And I have put in my memorial notes that I wish to have it played or sung.

This internal unexpected response to the verse and music is like a friend said to me: "A mystery to be lived, not a problem to be solved."

The music, which you can hear if you buy the CD, is often upbeat.

## The words of the music, "I'll Be on My Way"

*When I am gone, don't you cry for me, don't you pity my sorry soul;*

*What pain there might have been will now be past and my spirit will be whole.*

*I'll be on my way, I'll be on my way*
    *I'll have left my feet of clay upon the ground,*
    *I will be glory-bound, I'll be on my way.*

*When I am gone, please forgive the wrongs that I might have done to you;*

*There'll be no room for regrets up there, high above, way beyond the blue. When I am gone don't you look for me in the places I have been,*

    *I'll be alive, but somewhere else, I'll be on*
        *my way again.*
    *I'll have laid my frown and all my burdens*
        *down,*
    *I'll be putting on my crown, I'll be on*
        *my way.*

*"I'll Be on my Way" from the album "Meet Me on the Mountain" Used by permission. 2006 Shawn Kirchner Publishing (ASCAP)*
    *Sheet music available for order at www.ShawnKirchner.com.*

*A man's age is something impressive, it sums up his life: maturity reached slowly and against many obstacles, illnesses cured, griefs and despairs overcome, and unconscious risks taken; maturity formed through so many desires, hopes, regrets, forgotten things, loves. A man's age represents a fine cargo of experiences and memories.* ~Antoine de Saint-Exupéry

# Crossroads and Choices

*McFadden's notes on "Crossroads and Choices"*

*I have struggled with the decision about whether the following essay should be included.*

*It is very personal, and some readers may find it to be inappropriate material for a reflective book on death with dignity.*

*It is autobiographical, and yet there is no attempt to cover all of the details. In other words, it is not a complete memoir.*

*It is important to realize that this essay begins with a fictional ending of life.*

*For me, the pith of the story is not the details of the journey, but the reflections on belief.*

# The Time of Ending—
## Sometime in the Future

> *"I shall be telling this with a sigh*
> *somewhere ages and ages hence;*
> *two roads diverged in a wood, and I,*
> *I took the one less traveled by,*
> *and that has made all the difference."*
> *~ Robert Frost, poet*

I have often considered this time of ending. Some would say – this time of "passing," or time of "graduation." I have come to the present awareness that death can be simply a gracious time of ending.

When working as a chaplain in a Denver hospice, I was well aware of the dying of others. There must have been forty to fifty times that I was present at the time of the death of a hospice patient.

*I recall, with sadness, Edith*, an 89-year-old Lutheran, convinced believer, who came into the 26-bed patient care unit of hospice, ready to die. Very ready to die. And she did not.

She had uterine cancer, and it was terminal. And it was taking forever. Her heart was very strong, she did not go into a coma, and she was fully conscious and, unfortunately, alert.

She became verbally abusive—not to the nurses but to God. She was almost shouting at the Almighty. "Get on with it. I am ready to go." And then—when the ship did not sail and leave the pier as she had hoped—she was clear that God was not being fair.

She complained to me and to her pastor, "If He is so all-powerful, why can't He take me? I am ready, as ready as I will ever be."

Then one day, while the nurse was busy and was not paying close attention, she took a small scissors from the med tray and slipped it under her pillow. Later she attempted, very unsuccessfully, to cut her wrist.

Edith lived a few weeks longer, not in much pain, but not at all happy with God, her pastor, or the hospice chaplain. She drifted off one night, quietly. I can imagine she had a few words with the Creator.

*I loved Alex.* Not physically loved, though he was attractive. Slight, cinnamon-skinned, black wavy hair. I enjoyed his company. Only 21 years old. He was Hispanic, with roots in Mexico City. Gay and Catholic. He was on the count down and was going out with Kaposi's Sarcoma—at that time one of the many presenting illnesses of HIV/AIDS.

He loved his drugs, including alcohol, grass, and coke. He smoked whatever he could get his hands on. Robert, his partner, also had AIDS, and was also into drugs. Early on in my relationship with the two of them, they sometimes took me for an emotional and financial ride.

For instance, Alex would ask: "Could I borrow $60.00? We have to pay our rent tomorrow. We will receive our disability check in two days, and then we will pay you back." I knew better, but I allowed myself to be talked into making the "loan" because I was soft-hearted—and I liked him.

Kaposi's Sarcoma was not nice. It was an aggressive, disfiguring, and painful skin disease, and, at that time, always fatal. Alex hated it. I remember the time Robert and I took him in his wheelchair to the Denver Zoo for the Christmas lights. It was cold, and he was wrapped in blankets, a heavy knit hat, and a scarf that kept him from the very cold winds, but also covered most of the purple-colored facial blemishes. He hated the ugly-looking scab-like blotches. In the final days, he died not of KS, but of pneumonia—coughing and hacking his way into unconsciousness.

I was there. Later, as friend and chaplain, I conducted his memorial service.

Actually, there were two memorial services. His mother had one in his hometown in southern Colorado. The story for the family and friends in that community was that Alex had died of cancer. And his mother made it clear that Robert was not invited to "her" memorial service for Alex.

The service I conducted was in the Denver Metropolitan Community Church, and those present included Robert, many friends, and some of the hospice staff.

Alex's story of being gay and having AIDS was one of many similar accounts as I continued to learn something about the bitter-tasting judgments of family and the church.

*Then there was Earl*—an older gentleman—dying in his home with hospice care. He was, because of the excellent care of his family and the hospice staff, always clean, refreshed, and for the most part, pain-free. Earl and I enjoyed each other's company, and often our time together was spent singing hymns.

When I asked Earl about how he was dealing with dying, he told me of his favorite family travel vacations. As they drove from place to place, if there was a by-way that he had not been on, he would take the car in that direction.

As he explained it, traveling was an adventure. If he had not been someplace, then it was a quest, an exploration, and he loved it. And, as he said, "I haven't died before, so I look at this as an adventure. I wonder what it will be like and what I will see."

That's some of their stories. If I could choose what the ending for me would be like, my fantasy would be something like the following.

I am lying in a hospice bed—a special bed that has been brought into our home. It is positioned by the back window of our house in the master bedroom and looks out over the backyard with the gardens and ponds. It is summer. The gardens are a dazzling bouquet of flowers: hyacinths, impatiens, coleus, begonia, geraniums, petunias, marigolds, and zinnias.

The largest of the three ponds is right below the window, and, as usual, I enjoy hearing the water cascading over the rocks in the falls that run into the 2,300-gallon pond. When I sit up on the edge of the bed, which I can occasionally do, I can see the 16 large and smaller Koi swimming leisurely around the water hyacinths and the lilies. The Koi—regular and butterfly—are a symphony of color: gold, red, black, black over red, white, spotted white, and brilliant yellow.

I love this view. A magnificent, oak tree shades a large portion of the backyard. Other trees—magnolia, Dolga crab, black cherry, and yellow delicious apple—also add to the deep green of the summer.

From my perch at the window I can see our numerous birdhouses on the top of poles or hanging on branches. Several hanging blown-glass 10-inch globes sparkle and flash in the sun. And there are several garden statues— the "peeing boy" made famous from Brussels, the bronze naked boy entitled "Boy with a Thorn," and numerous rock and ceramic pots and planters. With affection I cherish this view because it is, for the most part, the loving handiwork of my partner, Keo.

The bed sheets were changed a few minutes ago. I was given my daily sponge bath. I am very weak. I have a catheter, but, thank goodness, no colostomy. This year the ITP (Immune Thromcytopenic Purpura) has come back with a vengeance—for the 7th time—and it appears that this will be the last time, for my immune system is mostly broken down, and now I also have a bone marrow problem—multiple myeloma. It is a blood issue ... the result of the platelet depletion. Remarkable, for acute multiple myeloma is what killed my father. Not inherited. Just coincidental.

No, I don't believe that this is the way God planned it. In fact, I don't believe that God or a god has anything to do with it. I have not the foggiest idea of a godness or being in my life or in the world at this time. Not too many years ago, I would not have made such a statement, but I have been in the midst of transition in belief for the last few years.

Slowly losing weight, pale, a little jaundiced, a beard but very little hair on my head. Several dozen chemo treatments. And I am tired ... exhausted.

Recently I have chosen, just as my friend Chuck did, not to continue with more chemo. Even if it worked, it would extend my life for only a few more uncomfortable and painful months.

I have no plans for the next-life future. I recall that at least one of the faith beliefs of some Jews—now and in history—is that when death comes, so comes the end of living. Nothing more. I am very close to believing that when this life is through, then this life is through. I have no lingering hope that I will see my parents. And I don't seem to need such a hope or promise or expectation. The possibility of graduation is, at best, mystery.

Oh, indeed, I will live on ... in the memory of friends and loved ones. When, as a chaplain, I would conduct a memorial service, I had a favorite reading, allegedly from the Book of Jewish Common Prayer.

Following are a few of the verses from the poem "We Remember Them."

> In the rising of the sun and its going down,
> In the bowing of the wind and in the chill of
>   winter,
> In the opening of the buds and in the rebirth
>   of spring.
> In the blueness of the skies and in the
>    warmth of summer,
> We Remember Them.
>
> In the rustling of the leaves and in the beauty
>   of autumn.
> In the beginning of the year and when it
>   ends,
> When we are weary and in need of strength,
>   When we are lost and sick of heart,

> We Remember Them.
>
> When we have joys and special celebrations
>     we yearn to share,
> So long as we live, they too shall live, for they
>     are part of us.
> We Remember Them.

I have, as a hospice chaplain and as a companion of those who have died, talked with friends and with many others as they have expressed their deep-felt, heart-felt, soul-felt belief that God is with them, and that they are secure in that Presence now and in the future.

And I have interviewed a dozen folks about their own beliefs and about their mortality. The beliefs differed widely among the religious and the formerly religious.

I recall talking with Chuck. He was dying, and he seemed at ease with simply not knowing about his after-death future. I guess that is what I am feeling. I don't know what is next or even if there is a next, and right now it doesn't bother me.

I recall that a young friend I interviewed said, when he talked about mortality, that the one thing he feared most was non-existence. For me, if there is only non-existence, then, when death comes, so comes the end of consciousness.

What I accept is that I do not have answers. There is a mystery to so much of life and living. And that is fine with me. Perhaps that is what being an agnostic is—realizing that an acceptance that life, living, and even dying is a mystery.

One day, very soon, with the continual and compassionate care of my partner, some of my family and many friends, and with the managed pain care and skilled nursing of the hospice staff, my breathing will slow down, become shallow, and then, quietly, I will breathe my last breath.

*Two Final Thoughts*

In a recent memorial service of an older woman, the husband gave the eulogy. They had been married for over 55 years—perhaps not all roses and sweetness, but nonetheless, not bad. Many of his remarks underscored her remarkable faith. God had always been in the picture. Even in her last few days, she made it clear to him and to the family that she was ready to die, and she was looking forward to being with God and the loved ones who had died in past years. The very essence of her life was that extraordinary faith.

For a few hours, following the service, I was depressed. Her life, at least on the surface, was excellent. It was, in many ways, a joyous occasion. We heard stories. We laughed. And many folks wiped away tears. But why was I so despondent?

Then I knew. I was envious. A recent reading of Michael Krasny's "Spiritual Envy, An Agnostic's Quest" suddenly became reality for me. I was almost overwhelmed with envy. I was hungry for what she had as an integral part of her daily life.

But in the hours that followed, I realized that I will likely, though I may be open to new insights, not ever have such a stable faith perspective that is dedicated to a god. Krasny makes it clear that the agnostic may choose to be open to new light but has also chosen that most of life is simply mystery.

So it is with me.

A second thought: I am responsible for this journey. I have made some of the choices. There have been crossroads. Yes, with no doubt, some of the choices have been unconsciously affected by the cultural climate and environment that surrounds and encircles me. I believe that much of the choice-making is a part of the incomprehensible mystery of life on this planet. Is it arrogant to suggest that I am entirely responsible for the choices that have been made?

Audaciously, I close with the familiar verses from "Invictus" by the English poet, William Ernest Henley. It is said that he wrote this poem as a demonstration of his resilience following the amputation of his foot due to tubercular infection.
I identify with his life reflection:

Out of the night that covers me,
Black as the pit from pole to pole,
I thank whatever gods may be
For my unconquerable soul.

It matters not how strait the gate,
How charged with punishments the scroll,
I am the master of my fate:
I am the captain of my soul.

# Part V

"Life should not be a journey to the grave with the intention of arriving safely in a pretty and well-preserved body, but rather to skid in broadside in a cloud of smoke, thoroughly used up, totally worn out, and loudly proclaiming "Wow! What a Ride!"

— Hunter S. Thompson, <u>The Proud Highway: Saga of a Desperate Southern Gentleman, 1955-1967</u>

# Appendix

## Resources

I suggest five books that focus on the 'death with dignity' theme. These books have been of great significance and importance to me in my thinking and writing.

### ** The Art of Dying Well: A Practical Guide to a Good End of Life
Katy Butler

"A common sense path to define what a 'good' death looks like" (*USA TODAY*), *The Art of Dying Well* is about living as well as possible for as long as possible and adapting successfully to change. Packed with extraordinarily helpful insights and inspiring true stories, award-winning journalist Katy Butler shows how to thrive in later life (even when coping with a chronic medical condition), how to get the best from our health system, and how to make your own "good death" more likely.

Butler explains how to successfully age in place, why to pick a younger doctor and how to have an honest conversation with them, when *not* to call 911, and how to make your death a sacred rite of passage rather than a medical event. This handbook of preparations—practical, communal, physical, and spiritual—will help you make the most of your remaining time, be it decades, years, or months.

Based on Butler's experience caring for aging parents, and hundreds of interviews with people who have successfully navigated our fragmented health system and helped their loved ones have good deaths, *The Art of Dying Well* also draws on the expertise of national leaders in family medicine, palliative care, geriatrics, oncology, and hospice. This "empowering guide clearly outlines the steps necessary to prepare for a beautiful death without fear" (*Shelf Awareness*).

## **To Die Well –
### Your Right to
#### Comfort, Care and Choice
Sidney Wanzer, MD 2007 and 2008

Knowing our rights to refuse treatment, and ways to bring death earlier if pain or distress cannot be alleviated, will spare us the frightening helplessness that can rob our last days of meaning and personal connection. Drs. Wanzer and Glenmullen clarify what patients should insist of their doctors, including the right to enough pain medication even if it shortens life. Everyone needs their wise and comforting advice.

> "Death ends a life, not a relationship."
> — Mitch Albom, Tuesdays with Morrie

## **Being Mortal – Illness and Medicine, What Matters in the End**
### Atul Gawande 2015

In *Being Mortal*, bestselling author Atul Gawande tackles the hardest challenge of his profession: how medicine can not only improve life but also the process of its ending. Medicine has triumphed in modern times, transforming birth, injury, and infectious disease from harrowing to manageable. But in the inevitable condition of aging and death, the goals of medicine seem too frequently to run counter to the interest of the human spirit. Nursing homes, preoccupied with safety, pin patients into railed beds and wheelchairs. Hospitals isolate the dying, checking for vital signs long after the goals of cure have become moot. Doctors, committed to extending life, continue to carry out devastating procedures that in the end extend suffering.

Gawande, a practicing surgeon, addresses his profession's ultimate limitation, arguing that quality of life is the desired goal for patients and families. Gawande offers examples of freer, more socially fulfilling models for assisting the infirm and dependent elderly, and he explores the varieties of hospice care to demonstrate that a person's last weeks or months may be rich and dignified. Full of eye-opening research and riveting storytelling, *Being Mortal* asserts that medicine can comfort and enhance our experience even to the end, providing not only a good life but also a good end.

## **Staring at the Sun: Overcoming the Dread of Death**
2008 and 2011
Irwin D Yalom

Written in Irv Yalom's inimitable story-telling style *Staring at the Sun* is a profoundly encouraging approach to the universal issue of mortality. In this magisterial opus, capping a lifetime of work and personal experience, Dr. Yalom helps us recognize that the fear of death is at the heart of much of our anxiety. Such recognition is often catalyzed by an "awakening experience"—a dream, or loss (the death of a loved one, divorce, loss of a job or home), illness, trauma, or aging.

Once we confront our own mortality, Dr. Yalom writes, we are inspired to rearrange our priorities, communicate more deeply with those we love, appreciate more keenly the beauty of life, and increase our willingness to take the risks necessary for personal fulfillment.

## **Finish Strong: Putting YOUR Priorities First at Life's End

by Barbara Coombs Lee
and Haider Warraich

**From the president of Compassion & Choices, *the* guide to achieving the positive end-of-life experience you want and deserve.**

It's hard to talk about death in America. But even though the topic has been taboo, life's end is an eventual reality.

So why not shape it to our values? FINISH STRONG is for those of us who want an end-of-life experience to match the life we've enjoyed. We know we should prepare but are unsure how to think and talk about it, how to live true to our values and priorities, and how to make our wishes stick.

The usual advice about advance directives and conversations is important but woefully inadequate. This book describes concrete action in the here and now to help live our best lives to the end.

FINISH STRONG will guide you through:

* Finding a partner-doctor to honor your values and beliefs with humanity, deference and candor.
* Identifying what matters most as vigor wanes and stating your priorities.
* Having meaningful conversations with doctors and family about expectations and wishes.
* Staying off the "overtreatment conveyor belt."
* Knowing when "slow medicine" is the best option to maintain quality of life.
* Navigating home hospice, the ultimate healing experience.

Written with candor and clarity by a nurse, physician assistant and attorney who became a leading advocate for end-of-life options, this book can help you FINISH STRONG.

**Two more books to be considered by Ralph McFadden**

## **For Life is a Journey – Reflections on Living**

Ralph McFadden was married and raised two children. But in the mid-1990s, he decided that living with integrity meant living authentically, "coming out" as the gay man he was. In *For Life is a Journey*, author McFadden, a former pastor, denominational executive, and hospice chaplain, explores his own journey as he confronts the church's blindness to the damaging injustice of homophobia.

*For Life is a Journey* includes McFadden's reflections about claiming his identity as a gay man and "surfacing his soul." He is honest about the depth of grief and anger that accompanied the changes he was forced to make in terms of work, his marriage, family, and friends. Through stories, poems and reflections, he discusses the sense of betrayal and abandonment that he experienced when the church that had so profoundly shaped his commitments to peace, reconciliation, and justice, now rejected him. He recognizes the internal changes that have occurred as a result of his journey toward authenticity and truth. From the struggling, the discovering, and the exploring came renewal and rebirth.

## **Into the Next Chamber – A Journey Worth Considering

**Noted by several readers:**
         Exceptional, Provocative and Inspirational

"Into the Next Chamber, A Journey Worth Considering," was published in 2013. This author's expectation is that the reader does not approach the content critically about the style of writing, or the rational or logic for the conclusions drawn, the personal story telling, or the lack of biblical content. Rather, the point of view of the writer, while it may be arguable, will be the starting point for the reader or group members to consider and reflect on his/her own core values and beliefs. Hopefully, the reader will find the content helpful in that he/she will move with anticipation into that next chamber.

The overall theme of the book is on "moving into the next chamber." As written on the back cover: "It may be time for you to consider moving into a new chamber. This new chamber is one we approach not with dread but with anticipation. It is a journey worth considering."

The living Nautilus is fascinating! This sea creature repeatedly continues in its life's journey by moving into a new and larger chamber. Oliver Wendell Holmes writes of the Nautilus: "He left the past year's dwelling for the new … Stretched in his last-found home and knew the old no more." What a striking and challenging metaphor! In each moment, in each day of the years of our lives, we build a new chamber. We initiate the next step of our journey by courageously moving into that new unknown promise.

Some have described the meditations as thoughtful, with unusual and perhaps controversial belief content, and provocative yet inspirational. One person wrote "I was very impressed and overwhelmed with his powerful writing, sophisticated argumentation, and clear statement for the freedom of acting and thinking for human beings."

# Legal Aspects

## The American Public

The American Public wants medical aid in dying. About 7 in 10 Americans across three different surveys say they support the option of medical aid in dying. In a May 2017 Gallop poll, a September Lifeway Research poll, as well as a November 2014 Harris poll, support is strong among almost all demographic groups.

Medical aid in dying also claims majority support among people of different religious beliefs, people of all ideological views (conservatives, moderates and liberals), people of both political parties, and all races and ethnicities. Support has nearly doubled since Gallop first polled on the question in 1947.

### Update on Jurisdictions
Oregon (1994) - ballot initiative
Washington (2008) – ballot initiative
Montana (2009) - state supreme court
Vermont (2013) – legislation
California (2015) – legislation
Colorado (2016) – ballot initiative
Washington DC (2106) – legislation
Hawai'i (2018) - legislation
New Jersey (2019) – legislation
Maine (2019) - legislation

# Power of Attorney for Health Care

As part of the preparation for dying it is of great important that the you know your advance directives. Note, Barbara Coombs Lee suggests that most advice about advance directives is "woefully" inadequate.

A friend that I worked with at Denver Hospice was an excellent nurse – and his wife was slowly losing her physical strength because of MS. Together they talked about and decided what would be of importance to each one, in the event a terminal illness. They put together a clear and very specific Health Care document that described what he or she would want.

Listed below is the website for Illinois and a copy of a document for Health Care. I assume your state has a similar document. Or simple search Google for possible models.

https://www2.illinois.gov/aging/ProtectionAdvocacy/Documents/POA_HealthCare.pdf

# Illinois End of Life Options Coalition

**MISSION STATEMENT:**

The Illinois End-of-Life Options Coalition is a broad-based, inclusive statewide partnership dedicated to raising both awareness and support across Illinois for medical aid in dying for terminally ill people (also sometimes called death with dignity).

The coalition's goal is to authorize medical aid in dying and ensure that terminally ill people who want it can access it. Email illinoisoptions@gmail.com to contact the coalition.

The Illinois End of Life Options Coalition is a joint project of the national group Compassion & Choices, the American Civil Liberties Union of Illinois, and Final Options Illinois.

We have come together to make aid in dying a fundamental legal right, here in Illinois. www.illinoisoptions.org

# Final Options Illinois

Final Options Illinois was founded in 1986. Back then, the national organization for aid in dying was called the Hemlock Society, and hence our original name was Hemlock of Illinois.

Final Options is dedicated to achieving legal change, to make aid in dying fully legal and part of accepted medical practice, in Illinois.

Aid in dying is truly a matter of simple human rights, and it is a human right we most fervently desire for ourselves, for our loved ones, and for all humanity. We all hope that we have a peaceful death ... but too often that cannot be possible without aid in dying, without the right to cut our suffering short, in a peaceful and humane way, if our suffering has truly become unbearable.

815-366-7942 or 224-565-1500
1055 W. Bryn Mawr #F212
Chicago IL 60660-4692
info@finaloptionsillinois.org

## Compassion and Choices

Compassion & Choices improves care, expands options and empowers everyone to chart their end-of-life journey. We envision a society that affirms life and accepts the inevitability of death, embraces expanded options for compassionate dying, and empowers everyone to choose end-of-life care that reflects their values, priorities, and beliefs.

Across the nation, we work to ensure that healthcare providers honor and enable patients' decisions about their care. To make this vision a reality, Compassion & Choices works nationwide in communities, state legislatures, Congress, courts and medical settings to:

Educate the public about the importance of documenting end-of-life values and priorities and about the full range of available options.

- Empower every individual with achievable options, authoritative information and constructive advice for guiding their care and engaging with their providers.

- Advocate for expanded choices, secure and ready access to them and improved medical practice that puts patients first and values quality of life in treatment plans for terminal illness.

- Defend existing end-of-life options from efforts to restrict access.

It's our belief — and our experience since 1980 — that the path to change starts with the individual, which is why patient-centered care stands at the core of all we do. Learn more **about the <u>Seven Principles of Patient-Centered Care</u>**.

800-247-7421
www.compassionandchoices.org

## *Compassion and Choices* - *Story, Focus, and Mission*

The nation's first Death with Dignity Act, co-authored by Compassion & Choices President Barbara Coombs Lee, was affirmed by an Oregon ballot initiative in 1994. Barbara was the chief spokesperson for this monumental law through two statewide campaigns, in 1994 and 1997. The first authorized prescription for medical aid in dying was written in December 1997 by Dr. Peter Reagan, former Compassion & Choices medical director.

Twenty-one years of the Death with Dignity Act has positioned Oregon as a leader in end-of-life care across the country. Oregon doctors and hospice experts who have been key implementers of the practice are sharing their knowledge and experience with other states across the country that have recently authorized medical aid-in-dying legislation. The law gives mentally capable, terminally ill adults with six months or fewer to live the option to request a doctor's prescription for medication they can decide to take to die peacefully, if their end-of-life suffering becomes unbearable. The law took effect in Oregon on Oct. 27, 1997, marking the first such law in the nation. In addition to Oregon, medical aid in dying is authorized in California, Colorado, District of Columbia, Hawaii, Maine, Montane, New Jersey, Vermont, and Washington.

Oregon doctors, hospice professionals and pharmacists are lending their invaluable expertise with medical aid in dying to states that are in the process or have recently authorized the option. This expertise takes the form of staffing Compassion & Choices Doc2Doc and Pharmacist2Pharmacist national consultation phone lines, providing education and advice to peers in other states, and testifying in front of state legislatures.

"Oregon has led the way for the rest of the country in authorizing and implementing medical aid-in-dying legislation, so it is only fitting that it lead in efforts to educate other professionals to help other terminally ill patients access this vital practice," said Kristi Jo (KJ) Lewis, Oregon & Truth in Treatment Manager for Compassion & Choices. "Twenty years of data has armed us with knowledge that will help professionals in other states acclimate to the practice at a more expedient rate, which is vital for patients living out their final days with a terminal illness who are considering this option."

Medical experts like Dr. David Grube, national medical director for Compassion & Choices and a retired family physician in Oregon who has written prescriptions for terminally ill patients, are training the next generation on implementing the practice through residency and Doc2Doc programs. Dr. Grube stated: "Oregon has over 20 years of experience with medical aid in dying, with a tremendous amount of data that assures us of the value of this option. As the data shows, many terminally ill patients get tremendous solace from knowing they have the option of a peaceful death, even though most will not find the need to use it. I am working to train established and up-and-coming doctors on this practice because these laws spur conversations between patients, their doctor and their loved ones about all end-of-life care options, and as a result, better utilization of hospice, palliative care and pain control."

These efforts are focused on removing barriers to the practice among healthcare professionals and facilities based on best practices learned from 20 years of implementing the law in Oregon. Compassion & Choices is also seeking to expand awareness through its Find Care Tool, which it implemented in 2016.

Since 2017, 3,278 Oregonians have accessed the tool to find medical facilities, systems and hospices with policies supportive of patient decision-making around medical aid in dying, of which there are 40 facilities.

Compassion & Choices will continue to provide support and education to the public and medical professionals. Its bilingual Access Campaign will ensure that every eligible, terminally ill Oregonian who feels that medical aid in dying is an important option has access to the Death With Dignity Act.

# Death with Dignity National Center

Peg Sandeen, Executive Director
520 SW 6th Avenue, Suite 1220
Portland, OR 97204
info@deathwithdignity.org

The mission of the Death with Dignity National Center is to promote death with dignity laws based on our model legislation, the Oregon Death with Dignity Act, both to provide an option for dying individuals and to stimulate nationwide improvements in end-of-life care.

Death with Dignity National Center is a 501(c)(3) nonprofit organization that expands the freedom of all qualified terminally ill Americans to make their own end-of-life decisions, including how they die;
 promotes death with dignity laws around the United States based on the groundbreaking Oregon model;
 provides information, education, and support about Death with Dignity as an end-of-life option to patients, family members, legislators, advocates, healthcare and end-of-life care professionals, media, and the interested public; and
 mounts legal defense of physician-assisted dying legislation.

www.ingramcontent.com/pod-product-compliance
Lightning Source LLC
Chambersburg PA
CBHW021420210526
45463CB00001B/460